# WOMEN
## Menopause and Middle Age

# Vidal S. Clay

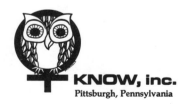

**KNOW, inc.**
Pittsburgh, Pennsylvania

Women: Menopause and Middle Age
by Vidal S. Clay

Library of Congress Catalogue Card Number LC 76-26455

International Standard Book Number ISBN 0-912786-37-X

Manufactured in the United States of America

Cover Design by Nancy Earle

First Edition, 1977

KNOW, Inc.
P.O. Box 86031
Pittsburgh, Pennsylvania 15221

# DEDICATION

To my father, Isaac Starr M.D., who, though he thought daughters would only grow up and get married, showed me by his own example that the life of the mind, of research and writing, was an exciting and rewarding one.

# ABOUT THE AUTHOR

Vidal S. Clay, Ed.D., is a lecturer in the department of Human Development and Family Relations at the Stamford branch of the University of Connecticut. She teaches two courses, Child Development and Personality and Marriage. She is a Marriage and Family Counselor with a small private practice.

Dr. Clay has published aritcles in professional journals: "The Effect of Culture on Mother-Child Tactile Communication," "Children Deal with Death" and a comparison of bereavement in death and divorce, "Where Are the Neighbors Bringing in Food?" She has also published articles in *Woman's Day, Redbook* and the *Single Parent*. She has a book in press at Watts Publishing Co., co-authored with Robert H. Loeb Jr., *Ms. or His, Your Right To Be You.*

Dr. Clay has lectured widely on the subjects of tactile communication, bereavement, and women, Women Alone, Being Single and Making It and Women, Menopause and Middle Age. She is active in feminist and women's affairs in Conn. She is a member of the local chapter of NOW and vice-president of Woman's Place, a resource center for women in Darien, CT.

Dr. Clay has been widowed twice and divorced. Her seven children are adult and independent. She has one grandchild.

# ACKNOWLEDGEMENTS

This book has been a serendipitous voyage. Several years ago I was asked to talk to a group of women on the subject of menopause. I replied that I knew nothing about it but after some reflection I accepted the invitation because I knew that I was close to menopause and although I didn't want to think about it, I knew I should understand it. My research went well, the talk was a success and the response of the women in the group was rewarding.

Meanwhile, I was changing my own head. I joined NOW and when I discovered the Task Force on Older Women, I joined that. Later I offered to write a position paper for the Task Force on the subject of Menopause and Middle Age. This book is the result of that effort.

First I must thank women. This book brought me back to women. Talking with women, sharing with women, listening to their struggles and worries, has made me glad and proud to be a woman. Special thanks to the feminists who encouraged me to write the book: Tish Sommers, of NOW's Task Force on Older Women, Marjorie Collins of *Prime Time*, Lollie Hirsch of the *Monthly Extract*. Thanks to the women who came to my lectures and afterwards shared a women's rap on menopause. Thanks to the women who wrote long letters expressing their feelings about personal menopause experiences. Thanks to the wonderful women at KNOW, inc., who put it all together: Anne Pride, Jo-Ann Evans Gardner, Felice Newman, Beth Kurlfink, Flo Scardina. Especial thanks to my editor, Beverly Stewart, for her insights and the confidence she gave me.

And much appreciation to those experts who gave me their help, especially Dr. Nathan Kase from the Yale Medical School, Sondra Gorney at the Center for the Mature Woman, Joyce Bockar M.D., Pauline Bart, Elise Maclay, Dana Raphael, Julie Lee and June Arnold.

Vidal Clay
Westport, Conn.
1976

# TABLE OF CONTENTS

# CHARTS

# WOMEN
## Menopause and Middle Age

# Chapter 1_____

# INTRODUCTION TO THE PROBLEM OF MENOPAUSE

*Menopause: A Normal Body Developmental Phase*

*The Effect of Society*

*The Climacteric: One of Many Changes*

### 1. MENOPAUSE: A NORMAL BODY DEVELOPMENTAL PHASE

The climacteric, or menopause, as it is commonly though mistakenly called, is a normal developmental phase in the life of a woman. Just as it is appropriate for a girl to begin menstruating in her early teens, so it is proper for a woman in middle age to stop menstruation. Unfortunately the normality of this physical and psychological process has been obscured by myths and taboos which reflect the ignorance, prejudices and distortions of our society.

## 2. THE EFFECT OF SOCIETY

A woman does not go through the climacteric, the years surrounding menopause, in a vacuum. Of course her body is affected by the physical process of the cessation of her monthly menses, i.e., menopause, but how she deals with this continuing development of her life is determined by her feelings about herself as a woman at this time in her life. These feelings will reflect society's notions about women, about women who do not reproduce, about women who are middle-aged and growing older.

Unfortunately women in this society are primarily valued for their youth and beauty, for their sexuality, and for their child-rearing and homemaking capacities. The time when a woman's menstruation ends is the time when she must face the fact of her own aging—and the end of her youth, her "beauty," defined largely in terms of sexiness in this society, and her child-rearing job. Menopause, then, is a Rubicon or crossing point, a "change" or a "change of life" which forces a woman to know she is no longer young.

## 3. THE CLIMACTERIC: ONE OF MANY CHANGES

The climacteric itself, however, is only one of a number of significant other changes a woman faces at this time in her life. Therefore it may contribute to making these years difficult. In order to understand why a natural and inevitable physical process becomes a problem to many women today, it will help to discuss it in its various parts—physical, social, and psychological—keeping in mind that they are all interrelated.

# Chapter 2_____

# THE PHYSICAL SIDE

*Introduction*

*Description of Menopause*

## 1. INTRODUCTION

The physical side of menopause is in some ways the simplest and easiest part of the problem for women today although it is the area women worry about the most. It seems obvious that women would find the climacteric easier to live through if they had accurate, factual knowledge about it. This information, however, is hard to come by. In reviewing the literature, very little was found to be known.

Historically, menstruation has always been a taboo area. Dr. Christopher Tietze writes about the relationship between negative attitudes toward menstruation and research. "This deeply ingrained interpretation of the catamenia (menstruation) as an unclean, unmentionable process has probably contributed to the neglect of the subject by physicians and research workers" (van Keep and Freebody, 1972). In the preface to a recent National Institute of Health pamphlet which is one of the best sources of menopause information there is, the editors acknowledge "a shared concern with gynecologists, endocrinologists, internists and clinical and research investigators over the lack of infor-

4

mation and data on the menopause as a total process in the human female" (Ryan and Gibson, 1973, p. vii).

Quite clearly, menstruation and its termination are female problems and as such have not been of interest to male physicians. The feminist joke comes to mind, "If men had the babies, abortion would be a sacrament." If men had menopause, it might be worth studying. (There is good indication that men have their own kinds of problems at middle age.) But it isn't only men who have this attitude. When a leading female sex educator was asked about menopause, she replied, "Entirely too much is made of it."

In no way can menopause be considered a small problem. In terms of numbers alone the problem is a massive one. There are 23.5 million women in the United States today around the age of menopause. One third of the women in the country are between the ages of 40 and 60. The National Institute of Health pamphlet points out that menopause and the climacteric are major factors in the health and well-being of a significant number of individuals (Ryan and Gibson, 1973). As a feminist and psychologist, this author feels that we need to know all there is to know about the climacteric and then the proper management of this transition period can be determined.

## 2. DESCRIPTION OF MENOPAUSE

In general it can be said that most women are in good physical health during middle age and into old age. Most women go through the climacteric with very little difficulty. Menopause is not an illness and you are not sick. No one ever died from it. Estimates of the number of women with "troublesome" menopausal complaints or symptoms range from 20 to 60 per cent. Despite the myths about the prevalence of emotional difficulties during menopause, many women, especially those who have not confined their lives to the wife and mother role, will go through "the change" with very little emotional upset.

Menopause is not the beginning of aging, because human beings age slowly throughout their lives. The aging process seems to accelerate after menopause, however. Menopause itself shouldn't make any great change in a woman's life. The only difference between a menopausal woman and a post-menopausal one is that the former is menstruating and the latter is not. The climacteric doesn't last long—about two years or possibly three for most women. Compare this figure with the average life span for women in America today, 75 years.

After menopause some women speak of a blossoming (Davidoff and Markewich, 1961). They feel better physically and have more energy. Other women report feeling more self-confident, more certain of themselves. Margaret Mead has called this positive change in women's attitudes and behavior which happens after menopause PMZ, for postmenopausal zest. In a recent talk she said she had observed "a post-menopausal zest . . . among women in almost all societies" (Mead, 1975, p. 498). Many women notice a smoothing out of their emotions now that the swings of mood associated with the menstrual cycle have halted. Physically there is a lessening of the problems previously associated with the menstrual cycle, i.e., premenstrual tension, periodic pains or cramps, irregular bleeding and overstimulation of the uterine walls.

Menopause occurs later than it used to, usually between the ages of 48 and 53, though it is perfectly normal as early as 40 and as late as 55. The idea that if menstruation begins early, menopause will occur late is a fallacy. The time of the climacteric depends upon a woman's heredity, her constitution and various environmental factors.

**Three Physical Changes**

There are three distinct physical changes associated with menopause. The menstrual bleeding ceases, the ovaries stop producing eggs, and the body decreases the production of the female hormones estrogen and progestin.

A woman's ovaries start to decrease the production of estrogen some years before menopause. Most women don't notice any change in their bodies until their late 40's when there are changes in the menstrual flow. The menstrual period usually tapers off in both amount and duration of flow although flooding occurs in some women. The periods may become irregular, closer or more widely spaced. This process takes from two to three years, after which the flow is ended.

## The End of Menstruation

A few women just stop menstruating. One woman reported, "I just woke up one morning and it was gone." It it likely that some decrease in flow had occurred though it wasn't noticed. "Sudden" menopauses of this type frequently coincide with some kind of upset—bereavement, moving to a new house or location, or serious illness (van Keep and Freebody, 1972).

## Not the End of Estrogen

Even though menstruation ceases, a woman's body still continues to produce some estrogen though it is not enough to build up the epithelial wall of the uterus and produce bleeding. In the postmenopausal woman the ovaries still synthesize small amounts of estrogen; also nonestrogenic material made in the adrenal glands is converted to estrogen at other nonglandular sites in the body. These sites are currently unknown. "These amounts may be clinically significant and can occasionally cause postmenopausal bleeding." (Ryan and Gibson, 1973, p. 10). Some women produce significant estrogen for as long as ten years after menopause; indeed, women produce some estrogen throughout the rest of their lives, though in minor amounts.

The important point to understand here is that "the change" is not a sudden shutting off of estrogen. In the climacteric the body has to adapt to less estrogen than it had before—that's why menstruation stops—but not to no estrogen at all.

## A Change in Hormonal Balance

Once the supply of estrogen is diminished and while the body is getting used to doing with less of it, a change in hormonal balance occurs which can lead to distressing effects or "symptoms" in some women. This period of hormonal disequilibrium can be understood as a withdrawal period. It is the same process as going off cigarettes, alcohol, or any drug on which the body has become dependent.

## No Two Women Are Alike

One thing the medical establishment agrees upon is that there is great variation in the way women experience this process of withdrawal. "No two women are alike," the doctors say. Some women experience a sudden drop in estrogen and develop severe symptoms which make them very unhappy (Connell, 1971). One woman in the author's menopause study reported that she felt like committing mayhem when she had hot flashes. Other women have a much calmer adjustment period. (For a description of the author's menopause study see Appendix 1.)

## Two Symptoms

The only two effects on the body which are directly attributable to menopause are vasomotor symptoms, popularly called hot flashes and sweats, and genital atrophy or thinning of the walls of the vagina (Ryan and Gibson, 1973).

**Hot flashes and sweats.** The hot flash or flush is defined as a periodic dilation of the small blood vessels of the skin. In other words, from time to time there is an increase in the diameter of certain blood vessels which allows more blood to flow into them. This gives the feeling of a rush of heat to the skin. It is often followed by sweating which, as it cools, can make a woman feel chilled. There may be shortness of breath.

**The variability of hot flashes.** The most obvious characteristic of the hot flash is its variability. Some individuals never have a single one. Perhaps four out of five women in early menopause have very mild flashes or none at all. For those who have them they vary in intensity, location on the body, duration, frequency and pattern. Medical writers describe the hot flash as a feeling of heat which begins at the chest or neck and sweeps upward over the throat and face. This description appears to be too limited. Hot flashes vary from Mild to severe. A mild one can be no more troublesome than a blush on the face. A severe one can be an annoying and uncomfortable experience. One woman described the development of what appear to be "severe" hot flashes as follows:

My hot flashes began as an intense itching and tingling sensation in my inner ear which came and went. When this began to wake me at night I went to an ear doctor. Neither he nor I thought to relate it to menopause. The periodic itching in the ears continued but it began to be followed by what I now recognized must be a hot flash. This would start at my feet and sweep up over my entire body in a wave of heat to my scalp. Sweat broke out along my hairline, on my face, chest, and rib cage. At night I would wake with a feeling of intense anticipation. I had time to take a complete breath and go into relaxation before a hot flash would begin. This seemed to help. After the flash had passed, I'd pull the covers back over me—thrown off in the rush of heat—roll over and go back to sleep.

At their worst I was having flashes like this every hour during the day and three or four times per night.

Hot flashes vary in location on the body. But no matter where they start—at the face, neck, ribs, waist or feet—they always seem to travel upwards towards the top of the head.

Hot flashes vary in duration. They may last only a few seconds or continue on for as long as a minute or two. Kaufman writes that the sensation lasts about as long as a labor pain, thirty or forty seconds (Kaufman, 1967).

Hot flashes vary in frequency from a few a day to as many as one an hour. They seem to occur more often towards the end of the day. They can be aggravated by anything which dimishes heat loss or stimulates heat production—exercise, eating, heavy bedclothes, warm weather, stress (Kaufman, 1967). They can be brought on by emotions. One woman wrote that she has them "whenever I feel put down as a woman."

**Hot flashes cyclic.** The overall pattern of hot flashes seems to be cyclic. They come and go. Speaking of the beginning of hot flashes, a gynecologist told me, "A lot of my ladies [sic] find that if you just do nothing the flashes go away." One woman reported that in the months she is menstruating regularly she has no hot flashes. When she has hot flashes she knows she won't be having a period that month.

It appears to be true that hot flashes are most common after menstruation is ended, but some women experience them while they are still having periods. In these cases there has probably been a change in the characteristics of the flow—less volume, more widely spaced, or whatever.

A 49-year-old woman went to her gynecologist for a six-month checkup. She reported that she was still menstruating every month and then added, "I'm having hot flashes." The doctor replied, "You can't have hot flashes if you're still menstruating."

Some authorities believe that women who are not having sex are more likely to have trouble with hot flashes than the sexually active woman. Several of my sample who were having both sex and hot flashes found no relationship. Mc-Cary writes that the more hot flashes a woman has, the less likelihood there is that other troublesome conditions will develop (1967). The author found no evidence to support this statement.

**Cause of hot flashes and sweats unknown.** Hot flashes are described as a vasomotor instability, but what actually causes them is unknown. Nor is it known why some women have them and others do not. It is well known that they respond dramatically to estrogen replacement therapy.

Hot flashes are temporary. In general they subside spontaneously even though the hormonal and glandular changes in the body persist. Once in awhile they return years later at times of emotional stress.

Hot flashes are annoying. They can be very uncomfortable. They can seriously interfere with sleep.

**Feelings of shame.** One factor that makes hot flashes especially unpleasant for women is that many women are ashamed of having them. One woman now in her 80's described an attitude that may still be common to women today. During World War II she was involved in important committee work. Sitting at meetings with men, she would feel a hot flash sweeping over her. She thought her discomfort was obvious "to all the men" and she hated it. This attitude of mortification about a natural body process seems to reflect the old-fashioned notion that menstruation is dirty and disgusting so it must be concealed. There is nothing inherently shameful about menstruation or about the symptoms associated with the termination of it.

**Hot flashes not obvious.** In point of fact, the hot flash is not as obvious to other people as it appears to be to the woman who is having one. Most people are unobservant. One of my subjects described feeling red as a beet and very embarrassed in public as the sweat poured off her. No one noticed. Of course she did not reach for a tissue and mop her brow, accompanied by sighs and groans emphasizing her terrible condition. Another woman checked her appearance in the mirror during a hot flash. After that she stopped worrying about it.

**Vaginal atrophy.** The second result of the decreasing supply of estrogen is vaginal atrophy. In some older women the tissues of the vagina become thinner and they do not lubricate as well. This condition can make sexual intercourse uncomfortable or painful.

Vaginal atrophy is always mentioned in the literature as one of the results of the climacteric. However it has not been studied. Remarks made about it are usually the personal observations of gynecologists. Many things are not known about this problem. For example, what proportion of women experience it? how long after menopause does it occur, five, ten, 25 years? what difference in occurence is there, if any, between sexually active and sexually inactive women? etc. Certainly the recent reports that sexual activity continues on into old age and that it is pleasant and fulfilling indicate that vaginal atrophy is not a problem to many women.

Further discussion of vaginal atrophy appears in Chapter 6, pages 87-93.

### Only Symptoms Helped by Estrogen Replacement Therapy

These two symptoms are the only ones helped by estrogen replacement therapy or ERT as it is popularly called (Ryan and Gibson, 1973). (There is some new evidence today that ERT may slow the development of osteoporosis, the condition of bone loss in older women, but the evidence to date is only supportive and not fully confirmatory.)

Right here on the issue of therapy or medication is where the physical, the social, and the psychological aspects of the climacteric interact most critically; the physical in terms of those women who have "symptoms," the social in terms of the notions that our society and the medical profession have about "the menopausal woman," and the psychological in terms of how the woman herself thinks and feels.

Before taking a hard look at what might be called the management of the climacteric, it will prove fruitful to see what our society says about women and middle age.

# Chapter 3_____

# THE SOCIAL SIDE

*Middle-Aged Women in America Today*

*The Postparental Phase: A New Problem*

*The Socialization of Women*

*Attitudes of the Medical Profession*

*Who Wants To Grow Old in America?*

## 1. MIDDLE-AGED WOMEN IN AMERICA TODAY

In the 17th century Sir Francis Bacon said, "Wives are young men's mistresses, they are companions for middle age and they are old men's nurses." At that time women's roles—the ideas about what women should be and do—were clearly defined for them by men and in relation to men. The same thing is true in large measure today, unfortunately, but how many women would accept for themselves the very limited and sexist roles described by Bacon?

### What Is a Woman to Be?

What is a woman to be in middle age, a man's companion? If you ask women what our society expects them to be and do in middle age, what would they say? Housewife? Worker?

Too old for a "sex object;" too young for a grandmother? A study of middle-aged college-educated women, who had living husbands and whose children had left home, found them answering the question as follows: "go to work," "be just a housewife," "society doesn't expect enough," "be a companion to your husband," "sit and get fat," "drink too much," "do good works," "play bridge and gossip," "nothing, absolutely nothing!" (Davidoff and Markewich, 1961, pp. 325-332). Certainly these women weren't sure what their proper role should be at this time in their lives, and their resulting feelings of confusion and anger are obvious.

**Lesbian Women and Middle Age**

There have always been homosexual women, sometimes called lesbian or gay women, who do not define themselves in the usual biological and social relationship to men. In America today homosexuality is still illegal in most states so homosexual women, like homosexual men, have had to keep their sexual preferences hidden. Recently the Women's Liberation Movement, by stressing the rights of all women to personal freedom, has begun to have a mitigating effect on the often hostile and fearful notions that this society has had about homosexuality. It is mostly younger women, however, who are involved in the social and political aspects of gay liberation and who are able to "come out," that is, acknowledge their homosexuality publicly.

Certain homosexual women today call themselves Radicalesbians. They refuse to accept the label lesbian for themselves as they feel it is a pejorative word used to put down women and to keep women in "women's place," i.e. subservient to men. The Radicalesbians call themselves instead "women-identified women." They believe that women must "begin disengaging from male-defined response patterns . . . if we are male-identified in our heads we cannot realize our autonomy as human beings" (Radicalesbians, 1970, p. 3). The Radicalesbians point out that a lesbian is forced to evolve her own life pattern, often living much of her life alone, learning usually much earlier than her 'straight' (heterosexual) sisters about the essential aloneness of life (which the myth of marriage obscures) . . ."(p. 1).

What are homosexual women to be and do in middle age? Are menopause and middle age any different for these women than they are for their heterosexual sisters? First of all there are usually no career changes for lesbian women in middle age. Most middle-aged lesbian women have been working to support themselves throughout their adult lives. Certainly in terms of paid employment they are likely to be in a good economic position for they are now well-established in careers.

What does a lesbian woman feel about the end of her menstruation? The end of the monthly menses will probably cause her far less sorrow than it does those women for whom reproduction has been a highly significant part of their lives. The pain that some lesbian women feel at the decision not to have children of their own seems likely to occur in early adulthood when they are struggling with the question of their own sexual identity. These feelings are poignantly expressed in a poem by Rita in the chapter on lesbians in the new edition of *Our Bodies, Ourselves* (1976).

What about the empty-nest phase of life? Some lesbian women have children, others do not. Those lesbian women who have children will face the same empty-nest or post-parental phase of life as straight women. Those without children will never be out of the job of child-rearing because they never were centered in rearing children.

Do lesbian women have different feelings about getting old than heterosexual women? It seems likely that women who have been searching for many years to find a definition of the self that is not dependent on a relationship with a man and which does not depend on accepting the traditional feminine role as the way to be female, will have less trouble accepting middle age and aging than straight women.

One of the tasks of life is to know yourself, to like and accept yourself. In this culture women are taught to identify themselves in relation to men—a daughter, a wife, a mother. Middle age is the time when a woman's children go off into the world, when her husband might leave too, and when she is faced with the aloneness of herself. Lesbians who have had to struggle and come to terms with the solitariness that is part of the human condition will most likely have worked out a sense of their own identity before middle age.

Of course lesbian women have relationships, sexual and otherwise, with other women. Close, intimate, sharing and rewarding human relationships are hard to make for any two people, and some lesbian relationships will pale and break up causing pain to those involved. Nevertheless the qualities that lesbian women define as attractiveness in each other seem not to be based to the same degree on youth, beauty and sexiness as they are in the heterosexual culture. If this is so, menopause and middle age are probably far less threatening to them.

The physical changes of the climacteric are the same for all women. The way women view these changes and other changes of middle age may be less difficult for lesbians than for straight women. Homosexual women have had different life experiences so they do not face so many major changes in middle age. Moreover they may have a more positive set of attitudes and values about the inherent worthwhileness of women. These feelings should stand them in good stead in middle and old age.

The advantages lesbian women may have over straight women in dealing with menopause and middle age do not indicate that the life of a middle-aged or older lesbian is thought to be an easy one. Older gay women continue to face many problems trying to live their lives in a society which is hostile to homosexuality, both male and female.

**Women in Magazines**

A search through recent women's magazines to see how middle-aged women were pictured turned up hundreds of pictures of lovely young women, some pictures of attractive children, but only one picture of a middle-aged woman. She was the stout, greying older woman in the mini-pad ad. "If you're going through a change (all this in darker type) the Stayfree Mini-pad will comfortably help you through the days when you don't know what's going to happen." (The advertising for this product implies that a woman's body leaks 365 days of the year from puberty through menopause.) In these magazines women apparently drop out of life at middle age.

One group of periodicals has plenty of full-page pictures of older women: the medical magazines. *And all these women are sick*, mostly with psychoneurotic (emotional) problems. Here are two examples. A full-page, full-color head and shoulders photograph of a sad-looking middle-aged woman set against a deep blue [sic] background. The advertising reads: *Premarin* (Conjugated Estrogen Tablets, U.S.P.) *Helps Relieve Emotional Symptoms of Menopausal Estrogen Deficiency Because It Gives Her Back Something She's Lost.* (The accuracy of this claim is discussed in Chapters II and VI.)

Another full-page color photo of a middle-aged woman's head, the woman looking pale and washed out. A medical hand is pulling down one eyelid to examine the eyeball. The copy reads: "The faces of iron deficiency anemia: one of them is due to menorrhagia (excessive menstrual flow)." The only place healthy, attractive and effective middle-aged women are pictured is *MS Magazine*. They had two splendid covers of Bella Abzug and Helen Gahagan Douglas.

## 2. THE POSTPARENTAL PHASE: A NEW PROBLEM

The question of what a middle-aged woman should do with the 25 or so years of living ahead of her is in point of fact a new problem. It even has a new name, the "empty-nest" or the postparental phase of life. There are three main reasons for this new problem: changes in life span, changes in patterns of reproduction and changes in patterns of work.

### Changes in Life Span

More women are living longer. It is estimated that there are about 27 million women over the age of 50 in the United States today who can anticipate living an average of 26 years beyond menopause. This increase in life expectancy is due, not to more women growing older, but to fewer females dying young. There has been an enormous decrease in the mortality of infants, children and young people.

## Changes in Patterns of Reproduction

The second reason for the problem is the changes that have occurred in the patterns of reproduction. In the past, and today in most parts of the non-Western world, most women bore children throughout the whole of their reproductive years, then died before the youngest child was reared. What this means is that the great majority of women in the world have spent their adult lives either pregnant or lactating and most have died young, what we would consider to be in middle age.

**Contemporary patterns of reproduction.** Today most American women limit their childbearing to a few years in their early 20's. This happens because many women believe that small families are desirable and because effective methods of birth control are now widely available and widely used. Statistics show that the majority of American women give birth to their last child when they are 27 years old. The result is that by the time they are in their 40's they have worked themselves out of the child-rearing job and are left with the children grown and gone and with no clearly defined, socially patterned and accepted "useful" work to do.

The fact that many American women have not had other productive work to do beyond housekeeping and child-rearing is very much a part of the problem of middle age. Looking at the years ahead after the children have left home, a woman may well feel "that devoting much of the rest of her life to domestic service for one adult male will keep her busy mainly with busywork" (Huber, 1973, p. 2). It is not surprising that when women are faced with the "empty-nest" phase of life, many of them end up feeling anxious, hostile or depressed.

One option for women in middle age has been to move into a second career of mothering when their daughters go to work and they rear the grandchildren.

In America the pattern of second motherhood is most often a working-class pattern. What has happened both in America and in Western Europe is that urbanization and increased mobility of people have caused this second motherhood to occur much less frequently than in the past (van Keep and Kellerhals, 1973).

The growing up of their children leaves a vacuum in the lives of many women. These women are not old. They are strong and vigorous. They have a third of their lives ahead of them without a clear social role to move into to replace the role of mother.

## Changes in Patterns of Work

Historically in America and in other cultures, housekeeping and child-rearing have not been the only or even the main occupation of women. In traditional societies generally, Oakley says, "the integration of domestic life with productive work life is a constant feature" (Oakley, 1974b, p. 13). All over the world adult women have done productive work like helping in the fields, growing vegetables, mending nets, making cloth, making crafts like lace or pottery for sale in local markets, working in a factory or a mama-papa store or whatever. For example, in the 17th century in England women produced most of the bread and beer. Women owned most of the beer-houses in London and the "ale wife" was a well-known character in rural areas. Brewing was important because beer contained essential nutrients. It was drunk at meals by everyone, children too (Oakley, 1974b).

In the Middle Ages marriage had an economic rather than a romantic basis. After marriage both women and men were expected to continue in productive work—agriculture, textiles or trade.

Consequently, there was no idea of the woman's economic dependence on the man in marriage; it was not the duty of the husband to support the wife, nor was it the duty of the husband to support the children . . . In practice the woman usually supported herself and her children through her own work. (Oakley, 1974b, p. 21).

(In fact, the old custom of women supporting themselves and their children is happening more frequently in America today, but neither the society nor the female heads of households are prepared for it. The results are severe emotional and social dislocations. The Census Bureau reports that 14 per cent of the children in this country are being reared by their mothers alone. Most of these women are the

breadwinners for their families as they are not being supported by the fathers of the children. Because of sex
discrimination at work and the low-level skills of most
women, this situation results in pushing these families into
poverty or welfare.)

To recapitulate, this is the first time that the majority of
adult women have been expected to make housekeeping and
motherhood a full-time job. Paradoxical as it may seem, this
cultural demand has occurred at a time when
technology—through household appliances and effective
birth control—has made it possible for women to spend much
less time at these jobs than was possible heretofore. The fact
that non-employed women today spend as much time in
housework as their mothers and grandmothers did, an
average of 55 hours per week, appears to be a matter of
socialization and choice, not necessity (Vanek, 1974).

In her review of the patterns of female employment in
America, Oppenheimer shows that before the country was
industrialized, most of the productive work was done by men
and women within the family situation (Oppenheimer in
Huber, 1973). In England, similarly, there was "domestic industry" which was work done and goods produced for the
exclusive use of the family, and there was also "family industry" in which the family worked together to produce
goods or services for sale or exchange (Oakley, 1974b).
Today domestic industry includes the unpaid work the
modern housewife does as a service to her family and family
industry has disappeared except for farm families. As society
became industrialized, most of this productive labor was
moved from the home to institutions outside the
family—shops, factories and the like. Because moving
women outside the home to work was thought to threaten the
stability of the middle-class family, it became the custom for
such women to take paid employment only in the years before
marriage. In 1900, for example, if a woman did paid work at
all it was in the years before she married or before the arrival
of children. At this time the proportion of women in the
work force declined steadily with age.

A change in the pattern of women's paid work occurred in
the 1940's with World War II when the great demand for

workers caused a decline in the prejudices against employing married or older women. The result was that the traditional pattern of women working outisde the home changed. "The first great departure was the entry or reentry of women past 35 into the labor force—those whose children, by and large, had reached school age" (Oppenheimer in Huber, 1973, p. 185). This pattern of paid employment of women over 35 has persisted so that today about one-half of the women between 35 and 60 are in the work force.

A second trend, beginning in the 1950's and becoming stronger since, is the increased participation of younger married women in the work force. In the 1950's only about one-fourth of the young married women (with husbands present) worked; today that figure is about 45 per cent. Furthermore, wives with preschool children began to take paid employment, as well as married women without children and those with children in school.

In other words, there have been major changes in the past 75 years in the patterns of paid employment of women from the days when only unmarried women worked outside the home to today when many women not only are in the paid labor force but also are working at different times in the family life cycle. Along with changes in the patterns of women's employment has gone change from negative to positive in the attitudes of society toward women who work for money.

What has been the labor force participation of those women who are middle-aged today? Women who are middle-aged now were in their teens and 20's when World War II broke out. After finishing high school most went to work while some went to higher education. After the war was over, most women, except single women, Black women and women married to poor men, left their paid jobs to become full-time wives and mothers. This was the period of early marriages, large families and togetherness. The few young married women who began to go out to work in the 1950's were far from typical of their generation. In the 1950's today's middle-aged women were busy producing the post-war baby-boom.

Today the problem of middle-aged women and the labor

force is that they grew up at a time when most married women did not work outside the home. They expected to make a career out of marriage. Women who have for 25 years devoted themselves to housework and rearing children and who have not had any other productive work to do are poorly prepared to enter the work force in middle age.

## 3. THE SOCIALIZATION OF WOMEN

The socialization of women in America has been dysfunctional as far as preparing them to do anything with their lives other than marry and have children. Most women are not brought up to be contributors to the outside world of work in our society. In her seminal article of 1964 Alice Rossi bemoans the fact that so few American women are engaged in *meaningful* work (Coser in Rose, 1973).

Because marriages are not arranged by families but are the result of the personal choice of the young people who have fallen in love, women are defined by their ability to attract men. The main thing a young woman learns in adolescence is to use "the cosmetic exterior of the self to lure men, find affection and succeed in the competition of dating" (Bardwick and Douvan in Gornick and Moran, 1971, p. 150). Girls are brought up to be weak, dependent and afraid of success (out of fear they won't catch a husband). This is the way they are prepared for marriage (Bernard in Huber, 1973).

Studies of women have shown that they have picked up the ideas about women that exist in our society. Even though people say they believe that our society is equalitarian women, and men too, show more respect for the achievements and qualities of men. "Too many women evaluate their bodies, personality qualities and roles as second rate" (Bardwick and Douvan in Gornick and Moran, 1971, p. 153).

Thus the majority of girls who were never taught or encouraged to be active, independent and assertive learn that they are important only when they are valued by men. A woman is not thought to be a complete human being by herself; she is believed to "need a man" to round out her existence. Women are taught to get their main satifactions in life from their relationships with men (and later their children), and they are expected to derive vicarious gratification from the achievements of their husbands (and children). Women are taught to live through other people. They are in serious trouble when the marital or love relationship falters, when they are left by men in separation, divorce, desertion or death, and when the children grow up and leave home.

There are a significant number of women who have resisted this patterning of women. Homosexual women have been struggling to determine a new definition of what it is to be female which is not based on the sexual and family roles assigned to most women. They are trying to find a sense of self, a centering of oneself on oneself, a sense of the whole person which is not in relation to men.

Some lesbian women try to find this sense of themselves in relationships with other women, thus copying the notions of the larger culture that personhood or a sense of personal worth can be found outside the self. Unfortuantely the cultural prejudices against age which are so much a part of the American culture exist to some degree among lesbians as well. Some middle aged lesbians lose their partners to younger women. When these relationships, sometimes called marriages, break up, the women experience the same suffering that "straight" women feel when they lose a man at the end of an affair, or through separation, divorce or death.

From the viewpoint of what we see happening in middle age to many middle class women, it is curious to compare the experiences of women who took different paths in life. Twenty-five years ago most young women married and settled down to raise a family. At the same time, some other young women, then considered strange or odd, began a serious commitment to paid work. Today, the women who did what the culture demanded may well be husbandless, and with their children nearly grown up and gone. Many of them are terrified of facing life for the first time on their own. Whereas the women who chose careers, either heterosexual or homosexual women, are possibly now well-established in their work and have made friends and a way of life that suits them.

## Problems in Marriage

The woman who gets married and settles down to live happily ever after by living through her husband and later through her children cannot have a truly satisfactory way of life. Back in 1949 when young women were rushing full-time into 100 per cent domesticity and the post-war baby-boom, Talcott Parsons wrote "it is quite clear that in the adult feminine role there is quite sufficient strain and insecurity so that widespread manifestations are to be expected in the form of neurotic behavior" (Bernard in Huber, 1973, p. 18)

**Marriage can make you sick.** Today we are learning that acceptance of the female role as it is defined in our society can literally make a woman sick. Vivian Gornick describes women as "outsiders," not really involved with the mainstream of life. She discusses the psychological cost to an individual of being "outside" (Gornick in Gornick and Moran, 1971). Jessie Bernard shows that although marriages are thought to be mainly for a woman's benefit—she's the one who "catches" a man—the "happily married woman" is likely to suffer from poor mental health. She found that married women are often depressed, phobic, full of fears, and passive (Bernard in Gornick and Moran, 1971). Pauline Bart studied middle-aged depressed women in a mental hospital. These women were the "good wives" who had not been aggressive and the "good mothers" who devoted their whole lives to their children. In middle age when their children have left, they felt useless and became bitter and angry at this payoff for all the years of being patient, hardworking and doing things for others. "Goodness" brought no intrinsic rewards. Those women "who move from the rigid wife-mother institution to the mental institution, are, in Bart's words, casualties of our culture" (Ehrlich in Huber, 1974, p. 270).

### Problems With Paid Employment

The way girls and women are taught to be, the kinds of personalities they develop and the hopes they hold for themselves relate directly to the kind of relationship that exists between women and paid work. For women, socialized as they are, paid employment cannot be very satisfactory.

The facts about women and paid work are stark. Today 35 million women work outside their homes. Women make up 42 per cent of the labor force; they make an essential contribution to the American economy. Most women work because they have to. Two-thirds of all working women are single, separated, divorced, widowed or married to men earning less than $7 thousand per year. "Despite the vital role they play in sustaining the economic well-being of themselves and their families, working women are paid 57 cents for every dollar a man earns" (*Women's Lobby Quarterly,* October 1975, p. 1).

This deplorable picture cannot be blamed entirely on the economic structure of American society. The way women are socialized and the personalities they develop are essential parts of this picture.

**The personalities of women.** How are the personalities of women described today? Here is the way psychological evaluations of women characterize them: inconsistent, emotionally unstable, lacking in strong conscience or superego, weak, nurturant rather than productive, intuitive rather than intelligent and, if at all "normal," suited to the home and family (Weisstein in Gornick and Moran, 1971).

These are not the qualities that lead to success in work in or out of the home, nor to high rates of economic reward in this society which equates success with rate of pay. In order to be successful in our society a person must show leadership, independence, assertiveness, judgment, and the capacity to take risks. These characteristics are not encouraged in girls.

With some exceptions, girls and young women are still begin socialized as though paid employment were going to be only a temporary or stop-gap activity in their lives despite the fact that today the average woman will spend 43 years in the paid work force (*Women's Lobby Quarterly,* 1975).

Komarovsky shows that even in an Eastern Ivy League college, women's attitudes about careers and having families haven't changed a great deal in the past 30 years. In 1943, 30 per cent of her sample expected to work for pay after the birth of a child; in 1971 the figure had doubled to 62 per cent (Komarovskyin Huber, 1973). This still leaves nearly 40 per cent of her high I.Q. college women planning to make childrearing and housework their permanent career. In a national sample of college-educated women taken in the late 1960's, 55 per cent of these women expected to get their lifelong satisfactions from marriage and the family.

A recent study of Angrist and Almquist called *Careers and Contingencies* (1975) describes the ways a group of college women make decisions about their adult roles.

. . . women in college begin very early to juggle the possibilities, to plan for the contingencies, of marriage and child-rearing and the other activities adult women engage in on an unpaid basis. A woman's life is much more built around these activities than a man's, for good or ill, and dedication to a full-time career often means turning one's back on pleasurable and satisfying aspects of life. What has looked like lack of ambition, aptitude or purposefulness in young women has actually been a very skilled and flexible figuring out of life goals, in which work plays a part, but not the greatest.

(From a review in *The Spokeswoman*, August 15, 1975, p. 7)

Mason (1975) did a survey of how women's attitudes toward sex roles have changed in the past ten years. Although it is concerned with sexual role stereotypes and not with attitudes towards paid employment, it does indicate that women's attitudes towards work are changing in the direction of a new recognition that paid work will be an important part of their lives. For instance, Mason found that in 1974 more women than ever insisted on equal job opportunities. Also, "an increasing majority, for instance, feel that 'a woman's job should be kept for her when she is having a baby' " (p. 520). This belief indicates an expectation that some women, at least, will want to return to work after childbirth rather than retire to the home and child-rearing. In 1970, 80 per cent of the sample believed "it is much better for everyone involved if the man is the achiever outside the home and the woman takes care of the home and family." Three years later, in 1973, agreement with this statement had dropped to a little more than 60 per cent. One of the greatest changes was in women's attitudes toward sharing the housework. In 1970 half felt that men should share the housework; in 1973 more than two-thirds felt this way. If the figures in these national surveys are really representative, it appears that changes may be coming for this generation in relation to women, men, housework and paid work.

**Work as a rewarding career.** What makes work satisfactory to the person who does it? Studies of men's satisfaction with their work shows that the proportion of men who like their work rises with the level of challenge, prestige and income they derive from it. It can be assumed that the same pattern applies to women. But in fact few women work at jobs that give these kinds of rewards.

Women's academic performance begins to fall off from high school on as they learn that academically successful and bright women may not get husbands. Once married and with children it is very difficult for a woman to continue a career. The realities of the burden of caring for small children shouldered by a young mother alone in her home or apartment without the help of other persons is such that it is the rare woman who has the energy left over to devote to the hard work and discipline that a career commitment requires.

Coser suggests that women "who choose permanent careers are expected to be likely to remain celibate, like Catholic priests" (Coser in Rose, 1973, p. 452).

The working-class woman is the one who most often will have to work for pay, but she is much more agreeable to staying home if her husband's pay increases than the middle-class woman. Some social scientists have described this behavior as lacking the motivation to work, but seen from another perspective, why would a woman want to be an assembly line worker, probably at less pay than comparable men, in addition to her work as housewife?

**The work that women do.** When women enter the work force they often continue to use skills they have developed inside the home and go into the kinds of work that require the qualities of nurturance, empathy and competence rather than the qualities of aggression and competition (Bardwick in Gornick and Moran, 1971). Half of all employed women are found in teaching, nursing, and secretarial or clerical work. Today women in the labor force are in jobs with low pay, low status or limited chances for advancement. No matter what job they do, women earn three-fifths of the salary of a man for the same job (Huber, 1973). This relationship between the pay of men and women is consistent throughout the Western world. The recognition of the economic discrimination against women is one of the main sources of the Women's Movement.

Rose Laub Coser's study of women and work brings a new understanding to the kind of work available to women (Coser in Rose, 1973). She describes how society assigns to men the primary role of breadwinner, and to women the primary role of wife and mother. Coser calls the family a "greedy institution" because it demands the total allegiance of women. Thus when a woman goes out to work it is expected that her work will be interrupted or disrupted from time to time by the demands of her family which the culture mandates as her primary commitment. Thus "women are in occupations in which each individual worker is *replaceable*, or *defined* as *replaceable*, and are not in occupations that are seen as demanding full commitment . . ." (p. 453). Coser takes public-school teaching for an example. For many years school teaching was almost entirely a female occupation. Behind the public-school teacher there stands an entire system of substitute teachers ready to fill in. (Coser points out that men disrupt their work for a variety of reasons, like going to professional or union meetings, performing special assignments for the government, doing research, or obtaining further training; these are defined however, not as disruptive but as part of the normal, acceptable and, indeed, professional work role.)

So it is that although 35 million women, constituting 42 per cent of the total labor force work for pay outside the home today, they are not expected to be committed to that work, for the culture demands their primary commitment must be to their husbands and families. Women's time is considered cheap just because they have followed the demands of the culture and put their families ahead of their jobs (Coser in Rose, 1973).

**Working two jobs.** Most women work for pay because they have to and others work outside the home to supplement the family income and obtain a higher standard of living for their families. Studies of working women show that most working wives not only work full-time but also do most of the housework. Husbands of employed women help very little more with housework and child-rearing than husbands of non-employed women (Cook, 1975; Vanek, 1974). This pattern holds true for Communist countries where most women work outside the home as well as for Western Europe and the United States.

How much time do women spend in housework today? In the past 50 years many household appliances have been developed to lighten the housewife's housekeeping chores. But at the same time, the nature of housework has changed with more time being spent in home-management, shopping and work defined as family care (Vanek, 1974). More time is spent doing laundry today than 50 years ago (ibid). Most people assume that women spend far less time in housework than their mothers and grandmothers did. This assumption appears to be false for women who are not employed; it is true for women who work outside the home.

Reflecting the lack of interest in "women's work" there have been very few studies of the time spent in housework. The studies that do exist show that women still spend long hours in housework. The term "housework" here includes all the time spent in housework, plus shopping and child care and supervision.*

In America, Vanek found that non-employed women spend an average of 55 hours per week in housework (Vanek, 1974). In England, Oakley found they spend an average of 77 hours per week. In France, in a 1958 study, the number of hours was 67 (Oakley, 1974a). Homemakers work longer hours than most people who work for pay.

How much time do employed women spend in housework? The International Labor Organization reports that working wives frequently work between 70 and 80 hours per week on housework plus outside paid employment. Assuming that these women work a 40-hour week, they must be spending between 30 and 40 hours per week on housework. Cook

---

*In case you have wondered how much extra work each child adds to a family, the French studies, which contain the most sophisticated breakdown of time spent in housework, suggest that on the average, one child adds 23 hours to housework time per week, two add 35 hours and three or more add 41 hours (Oakley, 1974a, p. 94).

studied working mothers in nine countries. She states that "homemaking-cum-motherhood often takes as many hours as does a paid job, and working mothers spend only slightly fewer hours at it than do professional housewives" (Cook, 1975, p. 28). American women have the most household appliances. (I was surprised to learn from Oakley's study that in 1971 English women "hoover" their rugs and some housewives are still doing their laundry in the bathtub.) Vanek reports that employed women in America devote about 26 hours per week to housework.

It is obvious then that the woman who works outside the home is carrying a double burden. She is in fact working two jobs: employment work *and* housework. The ILO comments that the key issue for working women is how to reconcile their home and family roles with their new occupational status.

Certainly for all married women who are in the labor force, some help and cooperation from husbands and children are important. Career women are described as having a "self-conscious gratitude towards their husbands for helping them to maintain a career" and for giving them the emotional support necessary to maintain two different and potentially conflicting roles (Feldman in Huber, 1973, p. 221). Davidoff makes the same point about the help middle-aged women will need in moving out into new careers. "Pioneering" is the term used and it is stressed that these women will need the help and support of their husbands and community in order to do this work (Davidoff and Markewich, 1961).

**Women and volunteerism**. Many women who do not have to work for a living undertake voluntary work in their communities. In this way they avoid the double burden of home and job and stay away from the competition, commitment, demands and frustrations of the labor force. By doing volunteer work, women get out of the isolation of their homes, have some adult contact, do some interesting work with social benefit, and have something to talk about at the dinner table other than the house and children. Someone described this work as continuing the mothering and maintenance work of the home by becoming part of the paternalistic institutional life of hospitals, schools, churches and synagogues (Gold in Gornick and Moran, 1971). Much good work has been done by women volunteers, and some innovative social programs have been instituted by women who saw a social need and had the freedom to meet it. A few examples are Head Start, sheltered workshops for the handicapped, recreation for old people, meals-on-wheels, tutors in English for non-English speaking school children, emergency telephone hot lines, welfare advocates, abortion and birth control counselors, work with prisoners to reduce recidivism, etc.

Feminists today are questioning whether women are not in fact being exploited for all the hours they contribute to volunteer activities. What may be lost sight of in this discussion is that the NOW statement on volunteerism was directed at service-oriented volunteer work. Volunteer work directed at producing social change was not considered exploitive.

Leaving these distinctions aside, the fact is that it is economically impossible for our society to pay volunteers for all the work that they do. Estimates of the number of people, men and women, adolescents and old people, who volunteer their services range from 37 million to 60 million. Chittenden (1975) writes that an estimated 60 million volunteers produced an estimated $50 billion worth of services. Our society has always depended on volunteers to make it work.

In her book, *The-Not-So-Helpless Female,* feminist Tish Sommers (1973) discusses the new spirit of activism that is appearing among women. She has three chapters on volunteers: Volunteers Beware, New Careers for Volunteers, and Volunteer Power. In these chapters she suggests how to stay out of volunteer traps like tea-pouring women's auxilliaries, envelope-licking, and neighborhood fund-raising which tend to keep women in their "place" and instead do what she terms "valid volunteering" in which you sue the system to gain your own goals rather than have it use you.

Today the number of volunteers is growing not declining. And there is an important trend towards training or professionalizing the work that volunteers do. It is being said that the skills acquired in volunteer work should count as work experience just as much as the skills learned in paid employment or the skills learned in school or college. Some women have successfully transferred the skills learned in volunteer work to professional work. Management skills and ability to communicate are essential to effective work in any area. Volunteer work has something to offer women.

## Problems at Middle Age

Women in middle age are faced with many changes in their lives and yet they have few options for the future. They were reared to marry and have children, and in middle age they find that the children have grown up and gone. And there are all those years ahead. What are their choices? Stay at home and care for one husband? Spend "his" money on clothes, cosmetics and redecorating the house? Take courses? Move into volunteer work? Move into the work force? Women who have stayed at home for 20 years are considered suitable only for unskilled work although some women who have done volunteer work use their experience as a stepping stone to paid employment.

Some women will be widowed at this time; others will be divorced. Divorce in middle age is a new trend. In the 1940's the divorce rate for marriages of 15 years' duration was four per cent. Today it is 25 per cent. A woman divorced in middle age is likely to face a difficult future. Because of her socialization she will probably look for another man but her chances of remarriage are slim. Moreover she is likely to have severe financial difficulties.

The new no-fault divorce laws have resulted in economic hardship for many women. Alimony is rarely given today and child support ceases, if it has been paid at all, when the children reach 18. In divorce these days women are seldom compensated for the years of unpaid work they spent as housewives. Women of 50 have few skills to sell in the job market and age discrimination, though illegal, is rampant.

This discussion of choices open to the middle-aged woman is biased in favor of the middle-class woman and applies only to those women who don't *have* to work for pay. For many single women, for women whose husbands are impoverished, paid employment is essential. The period of the climacteric comes and goes, but the pattern of life changes little. Many women had to seek paid employment while their children were in school; now that the children are on their own, they keep on working to support themselves. These are the women that Dr. Greenblatt of Atlanta had in mind when he said (talking about the treatment of working-class women with menopausal symptoms), "The woman from the lower stratum of society may not even notice that little bit of nausea and so for her stilbestrol is perfectly all right" (Chabon, 1973, p. 259). He was recommending a less expensive synthetic estrogen which has a 30 per cent chance of causing nausea.

## 4. THE ATTITUDE OF THE MEDICAL PROFESSION

The class prejudice and insensitivity of this remark are a good introduction to a final social problem that women have to face in middle age, the attitude of the medical profession. In general, doctors feel paternalistic towards women. This paternalism sometimes masks a deep hostility.

In terms of the climacteric itself, doctors often see women as sick rather than as passing through a normal body developmental phase. The disease model of medical education teaches doctors to think in terms of illness, and when a woman is "sick" the illness should be treated. This disease-oriented attitude causes problems for women in terms of all the natural female body processes, i.e., menstruation, pregnancy, spontaneous abortion and miscarriage, childbirth, lactation, weaning, and the climacteric.

Homosexuality is thought to be a mental illness in this society. The American Psychiatric Association recently decided that homosexuality should no longer be considered a mental disorder. Nevertheless, many medical people, and most lay people, still maintain the old views and many male and female doctors view lesbians as sick women who need to be cured. Because of this prejudice many lesbians hesitate to inform their doctors of their sexual orientation even though they need to tell their gynecologists that they are gay because it affects the treatment they require. One lesbian woman went to a gynecologist because she was having a bad hemorrhage. She had told him previously that she was gay but he kept insisting that she was having a miscarriage (*Our Bodies, Ourselves*, 1976).

Doctors, including gynecologists, have been found to be uncomfortable with, and uneducated about, sexuality. They are often made anxious by the subject of sex. Also their attitudes toward women tend to be stereotyped in the Freudian notions of femininity. It is not hard to see why women who tell their doctors that they are gay must often deal with doctors who are uncomfortable with this sexual orientation, who are often harshly judgmental toward them, and who are sometimes frankly curious about the details of women's sexual relations with each other.

The fact that many lesbians do not reproduce is a further problem for them in terms of their relationship with the medical profession. The male gynecologist's attitude toward women is reproduction-centered as reproduction is his main business. Lesbians, therefore, meet the same prejudices that face women who chose to terminate pregnancies, women who decide not to have children, or menopausal women whose reproductive lives are over. In addition, the prejudices lesbian women meet are exacerbated by all the other notions an MD may have about female homosexuality.

**Menopause—Disorder or Disease?**

An example of this way of thinking is seen in the description of menopause given medical students as "the most serious endocrinological disorder next to diabetes" (Ehrenreich and English, 1973, p. 76). One doctor called menopause a patho-physiological process, meaning that it is on the borderline between a normal and an abnormal process.

**Negative Medical Attitudes**

Another example of a distorted medical attitude is the way some doctors use the term "castrated woman" for the post-menopausal woman. This term can be correctly applied only to the woman who has had her ovaries surgically removed. Castration is an emotion-laden word for men as castration strikes at the heart of "maleness," the ability to have sexual intercourse and to impregnate the female. In whatever way men use this term for women, that is, accurately or not, what they are saying in effect is that a woman without ovaries or a post-menopausal woman is not a "real woman." Nothing could be further from the truth.

When doctors are talking professionally to each other, a hostile and deprecatory attitude towards women sometimes can be seen. At a conference on menopause one physician discussed the fact that at this time a small proportion of women develop an increase in facial hair. He called this "the Gilette syndrome."

A further pejorative medical attitude or belief is the one that says the menopausal woman is likely to have emotional problems. Dr. Howard W. Jones is quoted in a recent government publication as saying, in connection with the "psychiatric symptoms" of menopause, that menopausal women are "a caricature of their younger selves at their emotional worst" (Ryan and Gibson, 1973, p. 3).

**Medical education**

Diana Scully and Pauline Bart studied gynecology textbooks from 1943 to 1972 (Huber, 1973). They found that these textbooks were written from the male viewpoint. The books showed "a persistent bias toward greater concern with the patient's husband than with the patient herself" (p. 283). Here's an example of that attitude in practice. At a Boston roundtable on menopause the doctors were discussing the effects of an overdosage of replacement estrogen. One of these effects is breast tenderness and another is an increase in cervical mucus which leads to a vaginal discharge. Dr. Rafael Sanchez, a male, says that this discharge is pretty bothersome and asks the other doctors what they do about it.

"Dr. Greenblatt: I tell them to disregard it. It makes intercourse easier.

Dr. Irwin Chabon: I must confess to giving essentially the same speech. I hope you don't have it copyrighted" (Chabon, 1973, p. 266).

Out of eight medical doctors at this discussion, five were "delightful ladies;" not one of them spoke up to protest this point of view.

Moreover, in these textbooks traditional views of female sexuality and personality are still being presented "generally unsullied by the findings of Kinsey and Masters and Johnson" (Scully and Bart, op. cit., p. 286). Thus if a middle-aged woman goes to her gynecologist saying that she is not having enough sex in her marriage, a not unusual problem, how helpful will the doctor be who holds the outdated notion that passivity lies at the core of the female personality or who thinks that the male sex drive is stronger than the female sex drive?

Unfortunately many women accept the prejudices of the medical profession and of the larger society around them about women and about menopause. It is no wonder that they view menopause with anxiety and go to their doctors with complaints and "symptoms."

### 5. WHO WANTS TO GROW OLD IN AMERICA?

Who wants to grow old in a society in which the primary emphasis is on Youth? Who wants to be an older woman when there is nothing important for an older woman to do? The National Organization for Women is calling our society ageist as well as sexist and racist. In other cultures the accumulated experience of old people is respected; wisdom gets short shrift in America. (We wonder whether one measure of a society might be the way it treats old people.) Old people in America are encouraged to get out of the mainstream of life.

Old age is hard to face for both women and men. It is harder for older women because they often live longer, they often are alone, they often are poor, and they have more prejudice directed against them then against older men. It is no wonder that middle age and old age are psychologically hard times for women.

# Chapter 4 _____

# THE PSYCHOLOGICAL SIDE

*How a Woman Feels About the Changes of Middle Age*

*Menopause and Sexuality*

*The End of Mothering*

*Facing Middle Age*

*Facing Old Age*

*Changing Social Roles*

## 1. HOW A WOMAN FEELS ABOUT THE CHANGES OF MIDDLE AGE

The psychological side of the climacteric and of middle age is concerned with what a woman thinks and feels about getting older in this youth-oriented society. How she thinks and feels about what she will do with the rest of her life.

The first change a woman has to face is the end of her menstruation and the second is what that signifies. One woman in the author's menopause sample said to her doctor when she reached the climacteric, "I don't mind losing my periods but I don't want to get old!" It's this getting-old problem that makes accepting menopause so difficult for many women.

**The End of Menstruation**

For a lot of women the menstrual period represents youth and fertility, and the end of menstruation reminds them of the imminence and inevitability of old age. Helene Deutsch (1944) called menopause "a partial death." This notion may have been appropriate in the days when a woman was valued only for her reproductive capacity, but it certainly should be grossly inaccurate today.

**Feelings About Menstruation**

Psychologically women are believed to have a strong attachment to their menstrual flow. Van Keep points out a difference between the young woman who thinks "I still have time to . . ." and the older woman who thinks "there is no more time to . . ." (van Keep and Kellerhals, 1973, p. 161). Every month with the appearance of the menstrual period women are reminded that they are still considered young.

Women who are beginning to experience scantier flow and missed periods may feel sad about it; they mourn the passing of this part of their lives. Menstruation also represents being able to have children, and even though women would not choose to have a child at this time (one reason is the high incidence of mongoloid babies among older mothers), they hate to know that in a year or two they will have no choice at all. If physicians put women at this time on replacement dosages of estrogen and they experienced a menstrual type of bleeding, some will be pleased. Other women whose periods have ceased do not want to return to the monthly bother. If they take estrogens and have an artificially induced period, they will resent it.

Some gynecologists are keeping women on birth control pills until they are in their early 50's. These women do not know whether they are menopausal (in the climacteric) or not, because they are still having a regular monthly period caused by the estrogen in the pills. Like the women on estrogen replacement therapy, they too can feel they are still menstruating.

The wisdom of women taking birth control pills at this age and the propriety of women taking strong sex hormones for menopausal symptoms will be dealt with in a later section. The point to be made here is that the socially induced psychological need of a woman to think "I am still menstruating, I am still young" ties in with the need of doctors to give women something. As one doctor said about middle-aged women, "They feel better when they take a pill we give them."

## The End of Reproduction

Most women who choose to have families give birth to several planned and wanted children close together in the early years of their marriage. After that their reproductive capacity is a problem that has to be circumvented by the continuous use of effective birth control. Today one family in six is choosing sterilization as a permanent method of family limitation. This may be either a tubal ligation (tying off the Fallopian tubes) for the woman, or a vasectomy (tying off the vas deferens) for the man. Since so many women have given up their reproductive function voluntarily in their 30's, it would seem that the end of their menstrual periods should be much less of an emotional problem than it was to women in the past. For some women, menopause means the end of the bother of the monthly flow. It also means for many women a smoothing out of the swings of mood that ebbed and flowed with the 28-day cycle. And don't forget that PMZ (post-menopausal zest)!

Today the end of menstruation does not mean that a woman is old; it means that she is middle-aged. It does not mean that a woman is through with being a sexual person; it means that a woman is through with concern about the choice of bearing children.

## 2. MENOPAUSE AND SEXUALITY

In the past, menopause was equated with the end of sexuality. Sexuality was thought to be part of one's animal nature and the values of the time indicated that sexual relations were to be undertaken primarily for the purpose of reproduction or if need be to be a good wife and fulfill the marital obligation. Today it is recognized that sexuality continues to be an important part of the lives of both men and women well into old age.

## Sexual Interest Continues

Women do not become sexually disinterested after the climacteric. Sexual interest continues for a good many years until it begins to diminish gradually with aging. The need for sexual release becomes less frequent and the time it takes to reach orgasm becomes longer. However, the quality of the sexual communication may in fact improve as men and women have the opportunity to enjoy the delights of foreplay and the afterglow period, in a way that wasn't possible when the demands of youthful and inexperienced sexuality were more insistent.

Some women seem able to enjoy sex more after menopause when they are sure they can't get pregnant. (If a woman has no period for a year, she will no longer need to worry about conception.) It is the same sense of freedom many women felt when they first got the Pill.

## Women are Still Sexually Attractive

Women do not lose their sexual attractiveness at menopause. Jessie Bernard has pointed out that this is the first time in history that postmenopausal women are still sexually attractive. The middle class woman who has had good nutrition, good medical care, and who has not been worn out with superfluous childbearing and hard physical labor can continue to be attractive. Dr. Mary Calderone, an actress when she was young, and handsome now at 73, was giving a sex education talk to a school group some years ago. She asked for questions. One teenager asked, "How old are you, are you married, and are you still doing it?" Always very forthright, she replied "The answer to the first question is 64, and the answer to the other two is yes." She added, "Young people do not have a monopoly on sexuality. It is with you all your life" (Lobsenz, 1974, p. 8).

## The Persistence of Antisexual Attitudes

Still the old notions hang on and many people feel there is

something shameful and inappropriate about the sexual activities of older people. Older people themselves pick up these attitudes and they give rise to unnecessary feelings of shame and guilt about the needs for physical closeness and sexual contact that are a part of all human beings. A social scientist trained in the field of marriage and the family reported that after he and his wife became grandparents for the first time, he found that he felt awkward about making love to a grandmother. If his wife had been asked what she felt, she would probably not have had the same feelings. In our culture older men are considered sexually attractive and it is thought right for them to be sexually active much longer than women.

The contemporary idea that the sexual attractiveness of a woman is to a very large degree determined by the state of her physical body does great damage to older women. The psychiatrist and psychoanalyst Natalie Shainess writes about the disservice done to women by these attitudes.

Is there to be nothing left to share between men and women at the end of life? Why is there no appreciation for the contour of a woman's mind, as well as her breast. What if that breast's shape has been lost by nursing, or illness? Is that all there is to a woman? What if his fat wife is enormous—is she only the sum of her flesh? Could she have arrived at that state in an attempt to comfort herself because of his indifference? (1973, p. 10)

She continues that for older people the quality of the sexual encounter is what counts.

Men want, some say, to sleep with younger, firmer flesh. This is considered to be appropriate for them but inappropriate for women. If an older women does this, which she can do only if she has money and/or power, it is considered somewhat degrading (Shainess, 1973).

This preoccupation with the physical body of a woman makes difficult problems for women who have had certain kinds of surgery. An older woman reported that after her hysterectomy (uterus removed), her husband, a South American, refused to have sexual intercourse with her for some time as he thought she was no longer a woman. Women who have had a mastectomy (breast removed) are not considered desirable or even possible sexual partners by many men. Women who feel mutilated or worthless after these operations are to be pitied for they are reflecting the distorted attitudes of our culture. Shainess calls such attitudes obscene.

## Sexual Intercourse and Older People

There is the joke about the little boy who asked his mother, "Do you and Father have sexual relations?" His mother replied, "Why do you ask?" "I just wanted to meet some," was the reply. One of the problems of older people, older women especially, is just the same: how to meet some. As a woman grows older, the number of available men declines rapidly in proportion to the number of women. There are more than three times as many single women as single men between the ages of 45 and 64. In a singles organization like Parents Without Partners, which includes both divorced and widowed people, the ratio of women to men is three or four to one. In retirement communities the proportion of single, widowed, and divorced women outnumbers men 13 to one (Johnson, 1973). Moreover, some of these men are unavailable, either married or in sexual relationships of their own; some of them are inapproiate or undesirable; and some, of course, are unable. Masters and Johnson have shown that the end of sexual relations in middle-aged and older couples is often brought about by sexual incapacity in the male. One result is that certain women must either do without having their need for sexual stimulation and contact met or they must meet their own needs through masturbation.

Lesbianism is becoming more and more recognized as a possible alternative for some women. Phyllis Chesler (1972) believes that women have never been adequately nurtured by their own mothers. Women who move into relationships with women can get the nurturing they need, and give it too, within a sexual partnership.

## Masturbation, a Healthy Substitute

It is now widely accepted that masturbation is a normal, healthy and quite proper sexual activity for everyone from puberty to old age. Unfortunately the taboos about masturbation still persist and many older people are unable to use this sexual outlet or feel ashamed and guilty when they do.

The sexual faculty slows down with aging, as do the other processes of the body. To keep strong and fit one must keep active. The same principle applies to sexuality. The sexual therapists put it this way: use it or lose it. Masturbation is an appropriate alternative way of using it.

## Sex with Younger Men

Other cultures do not have the fixation on youth that we have in America. In France a woman is not considered interesting until she is past 30. A European male wrote a book, *In Praise of Older Women*, with the following dedication:

"This book is dedicated to older women
and is addressed to young men—
and the connection between the two is my proposition."

(Vizinczey, 1966)

## 3. THE END OF MOTHERING

By the time of the climacteric most women are through with their child-rearing responsibilities. A woman who had been happy bringing up a large combined family—his, hers, and ours—regretted to a friend that two of the children would be leaving home that fall. "Well," remarked the friend, "you wouldn't want them coming into the kitchen, lifting the pot tops and asking 'What's for supper, Mom?' the rest of their lives, would you?" The first woman had to agree; she really wouldn't want that.

### Time for the Children to Leave

The children have to grow up and go. Weaning is as much a part of mothering as is nursing. Levy and Munroe (1966) say "no mother ever delivered a child at adolescence with less pain than at the hour of birth" (p. 9).

The separation at adolescence is painful and many women mourn the passing of the children. They are not gone forever, of course, but a new type of relationship has to be developed now, no longer parent to child but adult to adult. For women who feel worthwhile only when they are mothers, the loss of the children is difficult indeed. Having nothing else to live for, some mothers won't let go of their children, causing severe problems on both sides.

Pauline Bart's study, cited before, of hospitalized, depressed middle-aged women, identified those women as "good mothers" whose only reward for years of sacrifice for their husbands and children was that the children grew up and left. Those women felt useless, "nobody needs me, nobody cares," and their anger at life took the form of deep depression.

A feminist who responded to the author's menopause questionnaire wrote that she thought menopause is "the time when a woman knows she has been had . . . and it's too late to do anything about it." (Hirsch, 1973). She was implying that our society dupes women into thinking that marriage and children are all there is to life. And when women realize they have been used, they feel very angry.

The emotional reaction to the empty-nest phase varies among women and it varies also with social class. Women with more education and higher social class have fewer physical complaints about the climacteric. This author's small pilot study found that college-educated women with high social class, high economic position and many interests found the climacteric little problem at all. Several of these women had late children. One mother of unplanned twins wrote, "They were the smartest thing I ever did." Women with late pregnancies do postpone the postparental phase, but whenever it comes it is likely to arouse feelings of loss and probably anger too, for it does require many changes in a woman's life.

## 4. FACING MIDDLE AGE

Menopause signifies to a woman that she is growing older. Middle age is part of life. First childhood, then adolescence, young adulthood, middle and old age.

### Be Your Own Person

Several of the women in the Davidoff and Markewich study described a blossoming after menopause. If a woman doesn't know who she is because she has always been somebody's wife or somebody's mother, it is a time to begin to learn. Middle age can be a time for self development and for getting back into the mainstream of life. One woman in the author's study described the freedom she felt now that her children were grown. She was widowed young and she had had to struggle hard. Now she felt that the job was done and she could live for herself. She felt a great relief.

The solution to the problem older women have of being active and productive, useful and happy for the next 30 years in an economic system which excludes them is absolutely critical to their psychological stability. In this society many women go straight from parents' home to husband's home and right into child-rearing without ever finding out who they are as individuals, as worthwhile people in their own right.

**No Clear Path to Follow**

At this time there is no clear path for women to travel in the postparental years of their lives for there are few generally known models to follow. Many middle-aged women will have to pioneer. As women are learning to create new social roles for themselves, it is likely they will feel anxious and disoriented at times. Some of the stridency of the women's movement reflects this unease.

Most women learn how to be women by modeling themselves on older women, mothers, teachers, etc., but each independent middle-aged woman striking out in new directions has to be her own model. Here is an example: After her 50th birthday—what a significant birthday that is—one woman pulled on a summer skirt which she had not worn for a year. It was several inches above the knee and it suddenly seemed very short—too short for a 50-year-old woman. "Oh dear," she said, "I don't know how to be 50 years old."

This problem with appearance may seem like a very minor disorientation, but it really is quite significant because the way a woman presents herself through her hair, clothes, body shape and movements is a reflection of how she feels about herself inside. The woman in the short skirt felt suddenly, What am I doing dressing in a short skirt when I'm 50 years old? *At my age* my mother wore skirts below the knee and stayed home taking care of my father and tending her rose garden. In fact, the confusion many middle-aged women experience embraces much more than dress. It includes attitudes toward self, life style, sexuality, paid work, etc.

## 5. FACING OLD AGE

If a woman is worried and anxious about growing old, then the effects of the climacteric will likely be more difficult and unpleasant than they have to be. In other words, if a woman hates growing older, then she will probably hate any discomfort from estrogen withdrawal she may have. This situation can be compared to the woman unprepared for childbirth who feels a hard labor contraction coming and cries, "Oh, God help me!" whereas the woman who has had childbirth education says when she feels a similar contraction, "Ah, I'll have my baby soon." In other words, what are horrible hot flashes to one woman who hates them as a signal of aging may be felt as nothing much by another woman who is not afraid or troubled by growing older.

### Menopause Accelerates Aging

How a woman responds to the notion of aging and to the process itself depends to a large extent upon what she thinks of herself as a woman. If she feels she is valuable only when she is young and pretty, then she is bound to have trouble with the climacteric and middle age. Women like this can go in for all kinds of reparative surgery, face lifts, eye jobs, nipple replacement. They can dye their hair and wear clothes in the latest style. They can shop around for doctors who will give them estrogen pills and promise to keep them young forever. They may be able to fend off the exterior signs of aging for awhile, but their denial of aging is really a hopeless game. Aging can be masked but it cannot be stopped. It is an irreversible process.

Women can be helped to grow old by seeing other women do it gracefully. When Elizabeth Taylor was 40, she is supposed to have said that she had earned every wrinkle on her face. She spoke with a certain pride about what she had been through. Woman whose mothers aged well have good models to follow. If we in this generation age well, we will help our daughters.

### Is Old Age Ugly?

Why do we think old age is unattractive in America? There is nothing inherently ugly about it; it is all in the way people think about it. The attitude that old age is ugly is learned.

A child may remember a grandmother who hid her hands in her lap because she said, she felt that the old age spots on the back of them made them look ugly. This was a comment the child could not understand since those hands put a cool washcloth on the child's forehead when she was feverish and those fingers played "painting fairy" games with her face when she visited at the seashore.

### 6. CHANGING SOCIAL ROLES

At the time of the climacteric a woman is likely to experience a number of significant changes in her life which affect the way she thinks and feels. It is likely that within a few years she will lose her own mother or father through death, she will see her daughter married and she will likely become a grandmother for the first time. Each of these life experiences will remind her that she is moving into the next generation. They bring her face to face once again with her own aging and with the fact of her eventual death.

Florence Rush (1971) writes movingly about the middle-aged woman in the middle who is caught between two generations. She points out that if a woman doesn't use the remaining years of her life for herself, she will never have another chance.

### Responsibility for Aging Parents

One of the psychological burdens of middle age is the responsibility for aging parents. Many people find it hard, once they have gotten free of the children and are looking forward to a few years of an unemcumbered life, to learn that they now have to take care of the parental generation. And it is hard, financially burdensome and emotionally painful. It is hard to switch roles and now take care of the people who once took care of you.

The choices that we in the middle generation make about the older generation, the manner in which we make them and how we carry them out may well influence how our children make these choices when we become the older generation.

## Becoming Widowed or Divorced

Many women will become widows in middle age and quite a few will be divorced at this time. Both death and divorce are hard on middle-aged and older women because the chances of going into the work force or of remarriage diminish with age.

## Making Friends with Women

Psychologically women have to deal with the fact that as they grow older there will be fewer men around. If women want friends they will have to learn to be friends with other women. Women who continue to live the way they were taught, as women competing against women for the scarce supply of men, cannot be friends with each other.

It is unfortunate that many women are prejudiced against women. Feeling second rate themselves, they don't think much of other women. One of the main values of the feminist movement has been that in it women have discovered that it is possible to like and respect each other. They have then been able to generalize to all women this tendency to like and respect women. As the anthropologist Dana Raphael (1975) says, one of the important effects of the Movement may be this giving women back to women.

When this author speaks to women about menopause I say that, as a single middle-aged woman, I've been looking for some mature men but the only mature men I can find are women. This always gets a laugh but it does serve to point up the fact that our society tends to produce mature women and immature men. If a middle-aged woman wants to find companionship, friendship, interesting and stimulating people, it is more likely that these people will be women than men.

## Facing Your Own Death

Middle age is a good time for women to make peace with their own death and dying. Many women of this age have already lost husbands or friends from cancer or heart attacks. Some women will die in middle age. Life is always chancy. It is easier to make peace with dying if a woman has become her own person, if she's done her own thing and fulfilled some of her own aspirations. If a woman has lived well and fully, it is easier to let go of life.

Life is a matter of loving and losing, and this is particularly a feminine experience. Little girls love their fathers and have to give them up to their mothers. Childbirth is a separation experience; some women have postpartum depressions. What mother hasn't grieved at her child's first day of school or when the oldest, and the youngest, too, go off to college? Around this time may come the death of parents. Women need to know how to separate, how to grieve. Accepting your own mortality is another separation process. Women do a lot of separating in their lives (Clay, 1974, 1975). Perhaps this is why they are said to die better than men.

Kaufman (1967) has pointed out that the climacteric comes at a bad time in a woman's life, a time when a woman is facing many major changes. If for example a woman's son is into drugs in college, her daughter is premaritally pregnant, her mother has had a stroke and has come to live with them, her husband is having an affair, *and* the woman is having to face the fact that she is growing older and life is passing her by, the physical side effects of the menopause may just be more than she can take!

# Chapter 5 _____

# ESTROGEN REPLACEMENT THERAPY

*Fountain of Eternal Youth?*

*Consider the Facts*

*Misinformation Abounds*

*ERT and Heart Attacks*

*ERT and Bone Loss*

*ERT and Sexuality*

*ERT and Depression*

*ERT and Aging*

*To Sum Up*

## 1. FOUNTAIN OF ETERNAL YOUTH?

People have always searched for a fountain of eternal youth, and Robert A. Wilson's (1966) ideas that estrogen replacement therapy would make women ''feminine forever,'' whatever that means, seemed to fulfill that need.

His book was reprinted both here and in Western Europe and the notion was spread to women by newspapers and women's magazines and to M.D.'s by the drug companies who stood to make large profits from this new medication. The result was that women went to their doctors in droves for this cure for old age. It was claimed by the experts, some of them financially supported by the drug companies who make the drugs, that estrogen replacement therapy or ERT would cure hot flashes and sweats, vaginal atrophy, stop the skin from aging, prevent heart attacks and osteoporosis (bone loss), cure feelings of irritability and depression and even increase libido or sexual drive.

## 2. CONSIDER THE FACTS

People believe what they want to believe. It now appears that only two of these claims are valid, and a third is questionable. Even more critical, however, the notion that estrogen replacement therapy should be taken by every woman from puberty to the grave as some doctors recommend, or from menopause to the grave as is advised by others, or just for several years to cope with problems of the climacteric, is very questionable indeed. In fact, *recent studies* (1975, 1976) *show a statistical relationship between ERT and the incidence of uterine cancer and breast cancer,* in women. Put more specifically, it now appears that women who take ERT are about seven times more likely to get cancer of the lining of the uterus than women who do not take it.

ERT is also life-threatening for those women with estrogen dependent cancers, as in the breasts, uterus, and ovaries; or for those individuals with arteriosclerosis (hardening of the arteries). ERT is certainly contraindicated because of the risk to life and health for other women due to family history, i.e., incidence of cancer and thromboembolitic disease (blood clots), previous medical history, i.e., cancer, high blood pressure, thrombosis, liver disease, diabetes, or because of the side effects. It is even highly questionable for the remaining women because the short-term benefits may not be worth the risks.

## The Two Symptoms Helped by ERT

To repeat: the latest medical opinion holds that the only two menopausal symptoms which are in fact helped by ERT are hot flashes and sweats and vaginal atrophy. Estrogen given in pill form by mouth—it is rarely given by injections today—is effective in stopping hot flashes. The thinning of the vaginal wall can be helped by application of estrogen cream.

## 3. MISINFORMATION ABOUNDS

Current medical opinion indicates that estrogen will not help prevent heart attack or osteoporosis (bone loss). In fact, taking estrogens may have the very opposite effect. Yet the myth that it will is still being published in medical and nursing texts, in pamphlets sold to doctors to be passed out to patients (*A Doctor Discusses Menopause and Estrogens* by G. Lombard Kelley, M.D., Chicago, Ill., The Budlong Press, 1959), in articles in the press ("Slowing the Clock of Age" by Rona Cherry and Lawrence Cherry, *New York Times Magazine,* May 12, 1974, New York, New York Times Co.), in collections aimed especially at women ("A New Look at Menopause" by Bernice L. Neugarten in *The Female Experience*, Carol Travis, editor, California, CRM, Inc., 1973; *Our Bodies Ourselves* by the Boston Women's Health Collective, New York, Simon and Schuster, 1973, 1976), and in popular magazines ("Look Better, Feel Better—Can Hormones Help?" by Dorothea M. Kerr, M.D., *Vogue Magazine*, January 1974).

## An Able Report

In contrast to this dismal record it is good to report that Joan Solomon's "Menopause: A Rite of Passage" in *MS Magazine*, December, 1972, offers a much more cautious and reasoned approach to the whole issue of medication and menopause.

## 4. ERT AND HEART ATTACKS

It has been thought that women were protected from heart attack and bone loss until after menopause. It was therefore hypothesized that adding exogenous estrogens (estrogens from outside the body) would solve these problems. This conclusion is now uncertain. Japanese women, Black women and poor women seem not to share in this. In fact, the "protection" that premenopausal women seem to have from heart attack may have nothing to do with women at all but relate instead to a curious vulnerability of the male to heart attack before age 45 (Furman in Ryan and Gibson, 1973).

In terms of older women and heart attack it is now known that, far from preventing heart disease, high dosages of estrogen may contribute to it because at elevated levels the female hormone estrogen has the effect of increasing the fatty deposits in the blood which is a predisposing factor to heart attack. In an editorial in the *Journal of the American Medical Association*, Dr. Nathan Kase compares the potential benefits of using estrogens at menopause with the risks brought on by this therapeutic intervention. He concludes, "Finally, estrogens increase the risk of thromboembolic disease, cerebral accidents, and coronary disease at high dose levels and in older age groups" (*Journal of the American Medical Association*, January 21, 1974, Vol. 227, No. 3).

Since the 1975 studies were published, women have been urged to be cautious about taking replacement estrogens because of the danger of cancer of the uterus, just as women over 40 are urged not to take the birth control pill because of the risk of heart attack.

## 5. ERT AND BONE LOSS

### Differences Between Women and Men

The bones of both men and women become decalcified with aging, but this problem is more severe in women than in men.

In both sexes peak bone mass is reached at about age 35, after which a plateau is maintained or a downward slope begins. The downward slope is statistically associated with menopause, and that rate of loss is greater than in men.

(Robert P. Heany, M.D. in Ryan and Gibson, 1973, p. 60)

The differences here between men and women are real. Women have about four times as much spinal osteoporosis (bone loss) as men. (Women live about seven years longer than men, so the effects of bone loss are more obvious among older women.) Hip fractures are about 2.4 times more common in women than in men. Forearm fractures in women begin to rise around age 45; by age 60, women have ten times the number of these breaks as men (*ibid.*).

### Estrogen Not Effective

In reviewing a number of studies in this area, Dr. Heaney reports:

Nevertheless, despite this veritable mountain of negative evidence, there still persists a notion that estrogens somehow stimulate osteoblastic activity in post-menopausal women, and are responsible for its maintenance in the premenopausal female. (p. 62)

He concludes his presentation by saying that estrogens have not proved successful in the treatment of osteoporosis and the efficiency of estrogen in preventing this disorder has not been determined. "Theory will not establish efficacy." (p. 66)

### Osteoporosis, Disease or Normal Aging?

In terms of osteoporosis specifically Dr. Heaney raises the interesting question as to whether it is a "disease" at all or whether it is merely the same as the ubiquitous bone loss due to aging. This question of labels is important because if the condition is determined to be disease, then the implication is that it should be "treated" in some way; and that a way should be found to prevent it. If it is understood as part of the normal aging process, then it will be dealt with in a different fashion.

## 6. ERT AND SEXUALITY

### The Popular Press

ERT is reported to be an aid to sexuality. An article in *Mc-Call's Magazine*, October, 1971, by David M. Rorvik, "You Can Stop Worrying About Menopause," has a lead paragraph about an unhappy housewife who reported that she couldn't stand to have her husband touch her, "intercourse was just too painful." But after taking female hormones all is changed, ". . . and now when my husband asks, he doesn't have to ask twice" (p. 102). *Girl Talk*, March, 1971, a magazine distributed to beauty parlors across the country, carried a piece by Dodi Schutz called "Have a Swinging Menopause." Everyone knows what the meaning of swinging is these days, sexual activity with a variety of partners. The main message in this article is, "Just keep the estrogens going" (p.31). *Harper's Bazaar*, August, 1973, had a section, "Bazaar's Over-40 Guide on Health, Looks, Sex." In it Jane Ogle wrote "Sex Begins at Forty."

Estrogen replacement therapy has come seductively to the fore. And what a little girl-Friday hormone it has turned out to be. There doesn't seem to be a sexy thing estrogen can't and won't do to keep you flirtatiously feminine for the rest of your days—and nights. It restores a feeling of confidence and well-being, makes your skin smooth and resilient, bounces up your hair, firms your breasts, sparks your interest in sex—a real package deal that spruces up your vagina, uterus and clitoris. In no time at all, everything is exactly as it should be: your whole body is primed for sex.

She ends this inaccurate and tasteless piece with the phrase, "So just lie back and enjoy it."

### Menopause Is Not the End of Sexuality

There is no basis in fact for the fear that menopause will affect a woman's desire for sex, her ability to perform sexually or to have full sexual response. There is no evidence that sexual behavior shows any radical change after menopause whether that menopause is a natural one or the result of surgery. Nor is there any evidence that hormones alone increase sexual drive in normal women (van Keep, 1973).

**Estrogen and Libido**

One of the rumors about the birth control pill was that it increased sexual drive in women. This result, if it ever occurred, was more likely due to freedom from worry about pregnancy than it was to the hormones in the Pill. Today depression and loss of sexual interest are both recognized as side effects of the Pill. In the book, *The New Sex Therapy*, Helen Singer Kaplan (1974) has a chart listing drugs which may enhance libido and sexual functioning. Next to progesterone she writes: "Does *not* increase libido, in fact may decrease sexual interest; acts on the cells of the female genitalia to enhance their growth, development and functioning" (p. 100).

**Estrogen and Vaginal Atrophy**

It is known that atrophy or wasting away of the vagina is helped by low doses of estrogens or by the application of estrogen cream. This therapy will help those conditions in which intercourse is uncomfortable due to loss of muscle tone and lack of lubrication of the vagina. Estrogen will help the mechanical aspect of sexual intercourse, making it easier to accomplish. It will not increase sexual drive.

**7. ERT AND DEPRESSION**

**Depression Not Infrequent**

Depression is not infrequently a concomitant of the climacteric in this society. Housewives have more depression than working women, and middle class housewives have more depression than working-class housewives (Bart in Gornick and Moran, 1971). However, studies of other societies show that middle age is not expected to be a difficult time for women. Therefore, emotional problems are not thought to be related to menopause per se though they may be aggravated by it. That is, anxiety and depression may occur (or recur) at this time, not becuase of the lessening of female hormones, but as a reaction to the individual's total life situation. Kaufman (1967) mentioned 100 women with depression and insomnia who were much improved on ERT; another 100 who presented the same symptoms were not helped. Of course it isn't known if the same results would have occured with the first group if they were given placebos, pills containing no medicine at all. (The fact that people do improve at least temporarily after taking placebos is well recognized. It is called "the placebo effect.") It appears that women who have coped successfully with other changes in their lives will cope successfully with menopause as well.

In point of fact there is an important interrelationship between the endocrine system and the neuropsychological system that women should know about. At the time of the menstrual cycle when women have more estrogen in their systems, there is a tendency toward premenstrual tension and depression. The estrogen in the birth control pill increases the amount of sodium in the body. High total body sodium has been associated with depression. Depression is one of the established side effects of the Pill. Although the strength of the estrogen in pills given for estrogen replacement therapy is far less than in the Pill, a depressed menopausal woman who takes ERT may have her mood lowered rather than lifted (Bockar, 1976).

**Attitudes of Physicians**

The attitude that women have toward their physicians and the attitude that physicians have toward their women patients meet here at the interface between menopause, women and therapy. It can certainly be hoped that Dr. Jones' expectations that women will be at their emotional worst during menopause are far from typical. Nevertheless, the notion that women will have emotional problems at this time is pretty widespread.

The attitude of doctors towards middle-aged women cannot help but be affected by the advertising of drug companies. Pictures of anxious, distressed menopausal women are used to sell both tranquilizers and estrogen medications. The implication in these ads is, Give women our products and we'll get them out of your office and make them easier for their husbands to live with at home.

Five years ago Robert Seidenberg made the point in his article, "Drug Advertising and the Perception of Mental

Illness," that drug companies by their ubiquitous advertising in medical journals and controlled circulation magazines, magazines sent free to physicians, are affecting or expanding the notions of what constitutes mental health or mental illness (1971). For example, the "treatment of choice" suggested by a drug company for the blues of an unhappy housewife are to start her on psychotropic (mind altering) medication, which may prove to be addictive, rather than to suggest that she try to cope with her life situation or change it or join a consciousness-raising group or whatever.

Today drug companies spend a billion dollars a year on drug advertising. Seidenberg estimated that they were spending $10 thousand per psychiatrist per year to promote the psychotropic drugs alone. Many physicians get their main education about new drugs from drug advertisements and drug company detail men. Doctors' ideas about sickness and health, and about women, so often pictured as "sick" in the drug ads, can be affected by all the advertising directed at them.

Moreover, the medical magazines are financially heavily dependent on the advertising revenue they get from their drug advertisers. Seidenberg suggests that their editorial independence, that is their ability to monitor improper or unethical advertisements for drugs, may be compromised by their financial dependence on the drug companies.

## The Doctor As Father/Therapist

It is tempting for doctors who see themselves as father figures to "these poor distressed women" in menopause to give ERT (and/or tranquilizers; one manufacturer now makes pills containing both medications) for emotional problems like anxiety and depression. Dr. Judd Marmor, a psychiatrist, spoke at a meeting on menopause sponsored by Ayerst Laboratories, the makers of Premarin, the leading ERT product. "Giving estrogen to the menopausal woman who is estrogen-deficient does more than merely replace a hormone. It is also supportive psychologically," he said (1973, p. 28).

It is not only male physicians who make an association between women, menopause and emotional problems. A recent roundtable discussion held in Boston on The

Menopuase and Estrogen Therapy was unusual because five of the eight participants were women (Chabon, 1973). (To date, women have been poorly represented or not represented at all at most conferences on menopause.)

In this discussion Dr. Lois R. Rollins reports that one of her standard questions to women at this time is, "Do you find your husband more bitchy [sic] and harder to get along with?" She continues, "And many times I have the answer, 'Yes, but how did you know?' So the actual change is in her rather than in him" (p. 244). Dr. Rollins is not aware of it, but she sets up the patient for the kind of answer she expects, and so finds that women are "bitchy" during menopause.

Later on, Dr. Ruth W. Schwartz brought out that some doctors give estrogen by injection because they feel certain patients need and want to come to the office "for that kind of social contact (if you can call it that)." She goes on, " . . . I discourage it."

Dr. Robert B. Greenblatt: "It's like going to church on Sunday."

Dr. Elizabeth B. Connell: "It's psychotherapy."

Dr. Schwartz: "There are other types of psychotherapy and that's not one method I use" (p. 261).

It could be wished that the distinction between female hormones and psychotherapy were as clear to all practitioners.

## TLC or Listen to the Patient

Earlier in the same discussion Dr. Connell gave voice to an attitude which, though patronizing, we wish were more widely held. Dr. Connell admits to using ERT in the treatment of mild emotional disturbances at menopause, but she goes on to say:

I think one of the most important drugs that you can administer is just plain old-fashioned tender loving care and reassurance. I think by and large this will cure many women. In my days as a general practitioner I discovered that half an hour exploring the life situation of the woman or what was really bugging her was sometimes a lot more helpful than the quarter grain aspirin you gave her as a placebo. I think it's the art of dealing with women and "what is your real problem" rather than giving her something empirically. One without the other is not good therapy in the long run (p. 236).

Gynecologists are among the busiest medical doctors. Some of them schedule their patients every 15 minutes. Few have time for a half-hour talk.

People who are anxious need to talk about their problems. Women can give each other the TLC (tender loving care) that the medical professionals do not have time for. Women can educate each other about menopause and so dispel the myths and misinformation that make menopause seem so scary. Suggestions for how women can become a support system for each other are discussed in Chapter 7.

### 8. ERT AND AGING

#### There Is No Cure for Aging

There is no cure for aging. Neither estrogen in birth control pills nor estrogen in ERT will keep a woman's body from growing older. Kaufman (1967) points out that women between the ages of 12 and 40 have large amounts of estrogen in their systems, but they still show aging.

Estrogen in expensive skin cream is ineffective in preventing aging of the skin. Some women put so much estrogen ointment on their skins to prevent aging that they have begun to menstruate again.

The popular idea that women can stay young forever simply by replacing estrogen is false.

### 9. TO SUM UP

Hot flashes and vaginal atrophy are the only symptoms of menopause that are helped by ERT.

# Chapter 6_____

# MENOPAUSE: HEALTH OR DISEASE?

*Menopause Not Traumatic for Most Women*

*No Complaints: No Drug Therapy Needed*

*Evaluating ERT: Benefits vs. Risks*

*The Medical Mess*

*Estrogen For Symptoms*

*Do Estrogens Cause Cancer?*

*Estrogen Replacement Therapy?*

*Estrogen Replacement Therapy—How Long?*

*Estrogen Replacement Therapy—
Does it Postpone Symptoms?*

*Conclusion*

## 1. MENOPAUSE NOT TRAUMATIC FOR MOST WOMEN

In point of fact, menopause is not the big trauma it is so often made out to be. Various authors report that between 50 and 70 per cent of women have no symptoms at all or only very mild ones. Half of the women going through the climacteric don't even go to their physicians. Of course, it isn't known how many of these women, if any, have complaints but think that putting up with discomfort during "the change" is a woman's lot.

Some years ago Jaszmann in the Netherlands did the only study this author was able to locate on the symptoms and complaints of the climacteric (van Keep, 1973). His sample included more than six thousand women between the ages of 40 and 60. He found the average age of menopause to be 51.4 years. From his data he was able to determine the percentage of women suffering from menopausal problems.

He grouped his respondents according to their menstrual age: those who still had their normal menstrual pattern (A), those whose cycle became more irregular but still had at least one menstruation in the last twelve months (B), and those who were in the postmenopause for one to two (C1), three to four (C2), five to six (C3), seven to ten (C4), and ten or more (C5) years.

He calculated then what percentage of the respondents in each group suffered from each complaint. In his opinion, only complaints which show a peak in one of the menstrual age groups should be regarded as a climacteric complaint.

His chart is reproduced on page 65.

It can be seen that hot flashes were the most common complaint and that they were experienced by a little more than 60 per cent of his sample. (The data do not indicate how mild or how serious the hot flashes were.) The chart clearly shows that the incidence of menopausal complaints peaks in the first year or two after menstruation has ended. After this period all the complaints diminish at a regular rate as the years pass.

This author passed out a short, anonymous menopause questionnaire at the 30th reunion, 29 years actually from graduation, of her college class. The sample was a small one, so the responses can only be suggestive. The college is a well-known, private women's (now co-ed) liberal arts college in the East. Most of the respondents were 50 years old. Twenty eight women filled in the questionnaire. Ten were premenopausal, nine menopausal, and nine postmenopausal. Two had had surgical menopause. A chart of their rating of their

**Chart I**

Fig. 1. Percentage of women suffering from mainly neurovegetative symptoms, defined by biological age.

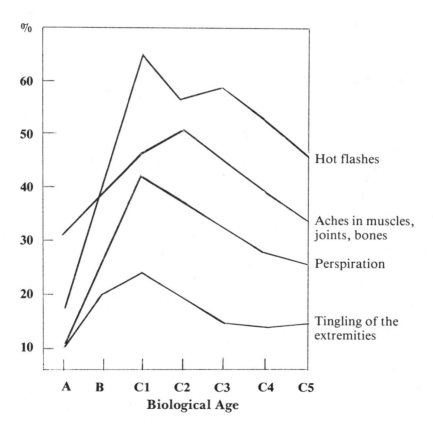

menopause complaints appears below.

| Symptoms | Pre-menopausal | Menopausal | Post-menopausal | Surgical | Total |
|---|---|---|---|---|---|
| None | 7 | 4 | 3 | | 14 |
| Minor | 1 | 3 | 3 | 1 | 8 |
| Annoying | 2 | 2 | | | 4 |
| Very Annoying | | | | | |
| A Real Drag | | | 1 | 1 | 2 |
| Total Subjects | 10 | 9 | 7 | 2 | 28 |

Half of the sample reported no symptoms at all. Eight had minor ones, four annoying ones, and only two rated their complaints "a real drag."

Seven of the postmenopausal women were taking ERT. Two expected to take it forever. Two had gone off estrogen replacement pills, one because she "couldn't stand it," and one because she developed fibroid tumors. Two women had surgical menopause, i.e., hysterectomies; one was on ERT and one was not.

The final question on the survey asked, What do you feel about your own menopause? Some of the responses follow: "It's been so easy, aside from a bit of depression, and I've been so busy that I haven't bothered to feel one way or another." "Passed without notice—true liberation." "It's for real! What I really feel is that *men* need more help. I've had lots." "Have been lucky as you can see from the above [had a child ten years ago]. "Glad it's over." "It's over, I think, and I'm glad, but it was far less bad than I had feared."

Menopause was certainly not a big problem to these well-educated, upper-middle-class women.

## 2. NO COMPLAINTS; NO DRUG THERAPY NEEDED

Almost all of the medical authorities agree, except for the extremists who believe a woman should take estrogen for the rest of her life, that unless a woman has "symptoms" there is no need for her to take medication. Kaufman (1967) states, "If you have no complaints and there are no objective findings of hormonal deficiency, no therapy is needed" (p. 57). In her report for Blue Cross, *Generation in the Middle,* Naismith (1970) says that the majority of women need no drug therapy at all.

## What Is a Symptom?

Menopause is a state of mind, an attitude, as well as a physical change in the body. The problem in defining a symptom is that what may be a serious complaint to one woman may be nothing more than bearable discomfort to another. The same hot flash that will be shrugged off by the woman who feels she's got everything going for her may appear intolerable to the woman who feels her life is in total disarray. One woman general practitioner who appears cautious in drug use said she felt that if a woman's symptoms were such that she came to the doctor about them, the woman should get hormonal therapy.

But surely such a rule of thumb is an oversimplification. It is no more reasonable than the rule of another gynecologist who would not give ERT for "minor complaints" but would prescribe them if a woman said her hot flashes were waking her at night [once? ten times?]. These notions about when to give strong drugs to women do save the physician the time and effort needed to make an individualized decision for each woman. It must be pointed out, however, that if the same patient with "symptoms" or hot flashes at night were given a half hour of the doctor's attention with an explanation as to what was happening to her body, how long it could last and what she might expect, she might decide that she is not "sick" at all but going through a normal body process. She would then feel very differently about the problem that originally brought her to the doctor.

## Physicians in a Difficult Position

It is obvious that physicians are in a difficult position. They are dependent on a woman's self-report about a symptom which usually cannot be examined in the office (unlike a sore throat or a broken arm) which they probably have not often observed in their patients and which they certainly haven't experienced themselves. They know that hot flashes are not painful, although they may be very uncomfortable, that they are not life-threatening and that they will go away in time.

Doctors want to do something to make people better. They know that ERT is highly effective in controlling hot flashes and until recently they did not realize that there were risks attendant upon taking the drug. Doctors need patients. Patients on ERT need regular appointments for physical checkups and for having their perscriptions filled.

To deal adequately with a woman who is full of anxiety about the changes of the climacteric requires a physician who has empathy, sympathy and time. One of the disadvantages of gynecological training is that doctors are taught that menstrual problems, and climacteric problems, aren't real; that they are "all in the head." So it is hard for doctors to get through the barriers and preconceptions of their education in order to meet the emotional needs of patients at this time of life.

Women are in a difficult position also. They are afraid about menopause and they are afraid about aging. They don't understand their bodies. They lack confidence in their bodies as a self-healing mechanism. Women have put their faith in the medical establishment; they believe doctors know what's best for them. They think that pills solve medical problems. They hear about and read about how ERT pills will solve their climacteric complaints and keep them from growing old, too. They want the medication. If they don't get it from one doctor, they may go to another.

**The Results to Date**

Since doctors have the authority and uneducated and unaware women are the passive purchasers of their services and of their medications, it is understandable why so many thousands of menopausal and postmenopausal women are taking these pills.

When the studies linking ERT and cancer of the lining of the uterus were about to be published in medical journals, the medical advisor of the Institutional Department of one of the leading stock brokerage houses wrote in a research report that in his opinion the results of these new studies would cause only a "modest reduction" in the sales of Premarin (Levine, 1975). He suggested that there would be some drop in the amount of pills sold, especially when ERT is used "on questionable indication" but he thought that in general doctors would continue to prescribe them and women would take them. He estimated a reduction of only ten to 20 per cent in the use of ERT for menopausal and postmenopausal women.

**An Informed Choice**

Certainly if women are going to take strong hormonal medication for the "symptoms" which occur as their bodies get adjusted to the decreased level of estrogen, they should be able to make an informed choice about this matter. The problem is that few clear answers are available.

## 3. EVALUATING ERT: BENEFITS VS. RISKS

Every individual who takes a medication should balance the advantage of the treatment against the risks that result from taking it. Estrogen replacement therapy is certainly no different; in fact, it is absolutely critical to make this judgment, because estrogen can be life-threatening.

The difficulties of evaluating ERT are four. First, up until very recently, no adequate long-term epidemiological research has been done on it. (So all the women taking it—and all those on the birth control pill—are in fact inadvertently serving as subjects in a massive study of the benefits and hazards of taking strong hormones over a long period of time.) Second, the topic is a complicated medical and chemical one, so it is difficult for lay persons to evaluate it. Medical opinions differ over interpretation of the facts. Third, many women have not yet learned to think for themselves. Fourth, most women have dependent relationships with their gynecologists or regular doctors. They will need to establish an equal partnership in which both parties discuss together what the advantages and risks of endocrinological manipulation will be. In short, what it means is that each woman must assert her responsibility for her own body.

## 4. THE MEDICAL MESS

### Wide Variety of Medical Opinions

Even though no adequate research was done until recently, physicians have been giving a wide variety of advice based on untested and unproved theories about menopause and the treatment for it. Within the medical establishment, *opinions* on this subject vary from what might be called conservative to extremist positions.

**The conservatives.** The conservatives see the climacteric as a normal part of a woman's life, not a "disease," which produces some discomforts in some women. These will pass in a year or two. They advise taking no medicine for hot flashes. Some will recommend a woman pay attention to her total health, diet, nutrition and exercise. *Prevention Magazine*, published by the Rodale Press, an organization devoted to the principles of organic living, had an article called, "In Menopause, Rely on Your Own Hormones" which stressed this point of view (March, 1970).

**The moderates.** The physicians who are moderate in their point of view suggest taking ERT only for the relief of symptoms. They recommend low dosages and going off the drug as soon as the symptoms have passed.

**The extremists.** The extremists believe a woman should take high dosages of ERT from puberty or menopause to the grave and they discount the problems that make other people cautious. Dr. Wilson's book, *Feminine Forever,* is still around and the Wilson Research Foundation, Inc. continues to circulate pamphlets like "Feminine for Life" (1964)). Dr. Wilson propounds his theories as if they were 100 per cent proven, but in reality they are a mixture of fiction and facts (van Keep, 1973). Dr. Wilson is not getting the support from drug companies that he once had because the Food and Drug Administration found his research unacceptable (Seaman, 1972). However, his pamphlet is still being distributed (May, 1974) by the Resource Center of the American College of Obstetricians and Gynecologists, which is very curious indeed.

The pamphlet states:

For the first time in history women may elect to avoid the physical and mental results of what is now recognized by the medical profession to be a deficiency disease—a deprivation of vital substances (p. 1).

All a woman need do to prevent the menopause—the results of estrogen deprivation—is to supply those substances the body is no longer providing (p. 7).

Supplanting from outside the body the materials it is no longer capable of producing is exactly the same type of replacement therapy practiced by millions of people taking, for example, thyroid tablets . . . . (p. 7)

Women are advised to take high doses of estrogen for the rest of their lives. This treatment will build up the endometrium or lining of the uterus requiring [an artificial] menstruation, a periodic "washing away" by means of five or six planned bleedings a year (p. 8, brackets added).

The Information Center on the Mature Woman, 515 Madison Avenue, New York, is funded by Ayerst Laboratories, the makers of the leading natural estrogen medication, Premarin. Sondra K. Gorney, the executive director, has published a book, *After 40: How Women Can Achieve Fulfilment* (Gorney and Cox, 1974). In it she says that "A lot of rough spots in menopause can be smoothed out by use of continuous estrogen medication" (p. 25). She goes on to say that taking ERT is "simply replacing an ingredient the body no longer is able to generate for itself" (p. 34). Thus she uses Wilson's opinions without given any indication as to her source. The book is in part, then, an advertisement for the product of the people who pay her salary. Nowhere is there any mention of the relationship between one of the co-authors and the drug company.

The purpose of the Information Center on the Mature Woman is to sell estrogen replacement therapy directly to women. They provide free filler items for the mass media. (As of April 1, 1976, they have discontinued their media service.) This is contrary to the code of ethics of the Pharmaceutical Manufacturer's Association (Seaman, 1972). The 1973 Annual Report for the conglomerate American Home Products Corporation reports on the division Ayerst

Laboratories as follows:

*Premarin*, the most widely prescribed oral estrogen, achieved a strong, steady sales growth in response to educational literature emphasizing its use for emotional disorders related to estrogen-deficiency. Greater recognition of the need to continue estrogen replacement therapy, beyond relief of the distressing symptoms which accompany the initial period of the menopause, has also aided sales (p. 5).

So the drug is now being pushed to aid "the emotional problems" of menopause and they suggest it should be continued even after menopausal symptoms have abated.

Premarin, with 95 per cent of the ERT market, is one of a number of prescription drugs produced by Ayerst Laboratories. $70 million worth of Premarin was sold last year. An estimated 1.3 to 1.5 million American women go through menopause each year, but figured from the sales of estrogen at least 5 million women are taking it (Cerra 1976).

When it is realized that there are 27 million women over the age of 50 in this country today, it isn't hard to calculate what vast profits lie in selling this drug to older women. It is typical of our profit-oriented society that the opinions of the medical extremists who push ERT as a panacea for the discomforts of menopause and the effects of aging have been the most widely disseminated. The conservatives do not command a large audience, and the moderates make no headlines as their reports are usually published in medical journals.

## 5. ESTROGEN FOR SYMPTOMS?

### Varieties of Estrogen

Estrogen is strong hormonal medication. There is considerable difference between the estrogen used in the birth control pill and that used for estrogen replacement therapy. Contraceptive estrogen is synthetic estrogen, an artificial petroleum-type chemical; the estrogen in replacement therapy is either conjugated equine estrogen, a natural substance made from the urine of pregnant horses, or it is a synthetic or artificial estrogen which comes in various forms. One of these is diethylstilbestrol, also known as DES, which is a coal tar derivative. DES is the drug in the "morning after" pill. (DES is now accepted as the cause of cancer of the vagina in the daughters of women who were treated with DES during pregnancy to prevent miscarriage.) Synthetic estrogen is much less expensive than conjugated estrogen, but it gives a higher rate of side effects, especially nausea. Although conjugated equine estrogen is a natural product, that is, it comes from another mammal, Pre-*mare*-in (Premarin), it is not exactly the same product as the woman's body produces.

Synthetic estrogen is approximately 60 to 75 times as potent as conjugated estrogen per milligram when the dosage is held constant. Thus a menopausal symptom which is helped by 1.25 milligrams of conjugated equine estrogen daily would require only .02 milligram of ethinyl estradiol, the estrogen used in contraceptive medications (*Journal of the American Medical Association,* January 18, 1971, Vol. 215, No. 3, p. 492). The various medications then can be compared only on the basis of the potency of the estrogen used rather than on how many milligrams of hormone there are in each dosage.

## Concern About Properties of Estrogen

**Estrogen a strong hormone.** Women have been concerned about the effects of exogenous (outside the body) estrogens on their bodies ever since the English studies on the birth control pill (Vessey and Doll, 1968) showed (1) correlations between taking the Pill and an increased rate of thrombotic vascular accidents (blood clots) and (2) that higher doses of estrogens led to higher incidences of thromboembolic disease. Since 1969 it has been recommended that women who take a birth control pill should use one with no more than .05 milligram of estrogen in it per day. The risk of death from blood clots in either the lung or the brain is approximately seven or eight times greater among women on the Pill than among women of the same age not on the Pill. Women on the Pill are hospitalized for blood clots about ten times more than women not on the Pill. In actual numbers the danger of death is slight. Three out of 100,000 women would die in a year from pill-induced blood clotting diseases. One in every two thousand would need hospitalization for a nonfatal pill-caused clot (Consumers Union, 1970, p. 5).

New research indicates that women over 40 should not take the Pill because of the increased risk of heart attack in older women.

As reported before, there is now strong evidence linking the estrogen in ERT to cancer of the lining of the uterus. There may be a link between ERT and breast cancer. Dr. Schmidt, Commissioner of the FDA, said in discussing replacement estrogens, "But the evidence is strong enough now for us and the American public to be on guard against the over-use, misuse and casual use of these substances" (Cerra, 1976).

In 1968, British medical sources reported an association between the practice of giving estrogen to women after childbirth to stop lactation (the production of milk by the mammary glands) and the incidence of thromboembolism (blood clots) in these women in the period after delivery.

A digression into the use of synthetic estrogen to stop the production of milk is included here because it is an example of the endocrinological manipulation of women's bodies by doctors who believe they are being helpful. Physiologically if a woman doesn't want to breast-feed after childbirth, her breasts fill up with milk and then dry up by themselves. Dr. Alexander G. Turnbull of Wales recommends "natural" suppression of lactation (the quotes are his) until more is known about the risks of estrogens. "Natural suppression is safe, practical and, in many respects, more efficient than stilbestrol." He goes on to discuss "natural" suppression in the following paragraph. The medical experience he reports here can be used to help women develop a new perspective on the problems they face in menopause. Dr. Turnbull:

Preliminary work has shown that although "natural" suppression causes some mammary discomfort in a minority of patients between the third and sixth days of the puerperium, this method provides subsequent freedom from mammary pain, recurrent lactation, and persistent bleeding—all of which outweighs the transient benefit of stilbestrol seen during the first few postpartum days. (*Ob-Gyn News*, May 15, 1969).

This example can be useful to women who have to decide whether to take or not to take ERT for the discomforts of menopause. It may well be that just as the natural suppression of lactation has proved to be the best, the natural suppression of the menstrual periods may also be preferred.

## Length of Time on the
## Birth Control Pill and on ERT

Women are concerned about how long they should take the Pill. It is now suggested that women take the Pill for a limited period of time—two, five, or ten years, depending on the doctor's opinion—and then go off it for a certain time in order to allow the body to return to its natural hormonal balance. Women can take the pill again later for another limited period of time.

Because vascular (in the veins) "accidents" occur more often in older women, women over 35 should be concerned about the dangers of the Pill. Because pregnancy is less likely at this time when fertility is declining, women over 40 should not use a birth control method which has a pill-related death rate for them of 25 per 100,000 per year from heart attack, strokes and blod clots.

The most popular ERT pill, Premarin, is taken cyclically like the birth control pill, 21 days on and seven days off. As has been shown earlier, physicians disagree about who should take it, about the dosage, and about the length of time it should be taken.

### Estrogen Equivalencies

The amount of estrogen in the Pill and in estrogen replacement therapy is quite different. Women taking the Pill take six to seven times the dosage of estrogen of women on ERT. The following chart is an effort to sort out these confusions by comparing the different kinds of estrogens available to women in terms of equivalent dosages. The chart begins with a column on the normal amounts of estrogen produced in the body of a mature woman. The footnotes are essential to a full understanding of this presentation. (See Chart II, pp. 76-78).

# CHART II

## TABLE OF ESTROGEN USAGE AND EQUIVALENCIES

| | Normal Woman | | Birth Control Pill |
|---|---|---|---|
| Dosage/Day | Ages 14-40 | .05 mg. to .5 mg cyclic | Synthetic Estrogen .05 mg$^1$ = |
| | Pregnant | 10 to 50 times more | recommended dosage for highest efficacy and lowest risk |
| | Ages 50 ff | Decreasing | Range of available pills = .05—.10$^2$ |
| Frequency | | | 21 days on, 7 days off |
| Duration | | | Not more than 2 years, 3-4 years, 10 years |
| Contrain-dications | None | | Poor blood circulation, blood clotting, clots in veins of legs, blood clot in lung, or eye, a stroke, heart disease, heart defect. Hepatitis, liver disease. Cancer of breast or reproductive organs. Family history of cancer or heart disease. Cystic fibrosis. High blood pressure, migraines. Diabetes if lactating; if over 35 yrs. |
| Side Effects | None | | Nausea, fatigue, breakthrough bleeding, breast tenderness, weight gain, fluid retention, headaches, rise in blood pressure, increased susceptibility to V.D., change in libido, skin pigmentation, depression, acne, gum inflammation. |
| Medical Supervision | 6 mo. to 1 year Pap, breast and pelvic exam; blood pressure. | | Every 6 months for Pap smear, breast exam, pelvic exam, blood pressure measurement. |
| Personal Supervision | Breast self-examination every month. | | Breast self-examination every month. |
| Cost | Medical appointments: $5—$30. | | About $35/year for the Pill. Plus cost of two medical appointments. |

| Estrogen Replacement Therapy (ERT) | | | "Morning After" Pill | |
|---|---|---|---|---|
| Conjugated Estrogen (Premarin) | Diethylstilbestrol (DES) | Ethinyl (Estradiol) | Diethylstilbestrol (DES) | Conjugated Estrogen |
| .3 mg—green[3] .625 mg—red[3] | .25 mg[3] | .01 to .05 mg[3] | | |
| 1.25 mg—yellow 2.5 mg—purple | 1 mg[5] | .05 mg | 5 mg | unknown |
| 21 days on, 7 days off | | | Twice/day | |
| Start it, then stop it to see results. Not more than 2 years—forever | | | 5 Days | 20 Days |
| Warning: ERT may cause cancer of the uterus or breasts. See comments at left, under Birth Control Pill. | | | Family history of cancer, irregular bleeding, maternal history of DES during pregnancy[4] | |
| Mastitis (lumps in breast). | | | | |
| ? in relation to previous use of birth control pill. | | | | |
| Caution: Women over 50[6]. | | | | |
| Break-through bleeding, nausea, breast tenderness, weight gain, fluid retention, headache, vaginal discharge, skin pigmentation. | | | Nausea and vomiting. | |
| See comments at left, under Birth Control Pill. | | | ? | |
| See comments at left, under Birth Control Pill. | | | ? | |
| Synthetic estrogen is less costly than Premarin. High dose, about $25/year; low dose, about $15/year. Plus cost of two medical appointments. | | | About $2.00 Plus medical visit. | |

# Footnotes to Chart II

1. In December,1969 the British Committee on the Safety of Drugs recommended to all British physicians that they prescribe pills with .05 mg. of estrogen. The FDA gave the same advice in the U.S.A.

2. The FDA estimated that about half the 8.5 million women on the pill are taking preparations that contain more than .05 mg. of estrogen (*Consumers Union*, 1970, p. 20).

3. The FDA is preparing warning labels linking ERT and cancer of the uterus. The FDA will probably recommend the dose be as low as possible and the drug be taken for as short a time as possible.

   Appropriate dosages recommended by National Institute of Health, equivalent to amount of estrogen a woman normally produces. No estimate is available as to how many women are taking the higher dose pills.

4. Diminishing use today since the relationship between DES and vaginal cancer become recognized.

   Over 100 cases of cancer of the cervix or vagina have now been detected in young women whose mothers took DES in the 1940's and 1950's to prevent miscarriage. This drug is still being used as a morning-after or postcoital contraceptive. Dr. P. Greenwald, director, Cancer Control Bureau, New York State Health Department, warns: "It seems likely that widespread use of DES as a morning-after pill will result in some daughters born with this vaginal cancer risk . . ." (Goodman, 1974, p. 8)

5. Will cause nausea and gastric upset in about 20 per cent of patients.

6. In this age group the appearance of vaginal bleeding must be differentiated from uterine cancer by repeated cytologic (cell structure) evaluations.

7. The use of DES as a post-coital or "morning after" contraceptive is now extremely controversial.

## The Risks

At this writing the FDA is drawing up a set of recommendations which will limit the use of estrogens for the treatment of menopause symptoms and aftereffects.

**Contraindications.** It can be seen by the chart that the contraindications for taking ERT are similar to those for the birth control pill. Women with a history of blood clots and those with a family history of cancer of the breast or cervix, or women who have had cancer themselves should not take estrogen replacement therapy. Women should not take ERT if they have irregular bleeding or benign (noncancerous) tumors of the breasts or uterus.

**Regular medical supervision.** Women who take ERT, like women on the Pill, should go to their doctors for checkups every six months for breast, vaginal and rectal examinations and a Pap smear. All women should do breast checks on themselves every month. Every woman on ERT should have her dose individualized by her physician in accordance with her family history, her previous medical history, and her special, individual needs.

**Side effects.** Like the Pill, ERT has various side effects. Ayerts Labs, in one of their advertisements for Permarin, state the problem of side effects as follows:

As with other medications, estrogen administration is capable of producing occasional side effects in susceptible patients. However . . . many symptoms abate or disappear with continuous administration. Among phenomena observed are gastrointestinal disturbances, fluid retention and weight gain, breast and pelvic discomfort due to tissue enlargement, headache, vaginal discharge and skin pigmentation.

One of the main side effects of ERT is so-called "breakthrough bleeding." It sometimes happens that small amounts of estrogen taken on a continuous or semicontinuous basis cause bleeding. The problem here is that it is difficult to determine whether this flow is due to ERT or whether it is a sign of something more serious, i.e., cancer of the endometrium (lining of the uterus). In other words, "breakthrough bleeding" or the normal "withdrawal" bleeding that occurs in women on higher doses of ERT can mask signs of cancer of the uterus. *Any spotting or bleeding in a postmenopausal woman should be checked by a physician at once.* After menopause vaginal bleeding is the most common symptom of cancer of the endometrium (lining of the uterus). If the disease is discovered early, it is highly curable by surgery to remove the uterus (hysterectomy) and by radiation therapy.

## 6. DO ESTROGENS CAUSE CANCER?

Today the practice of taking estrogens for the symptoms of menopause and postmenopausally has been firmly linked by statistical data to cancer of the uterus. At this time there is no conclusive medical proof of a direct cause and effect relationship between ERT and uterine cancer. However the statistical relationship should be taken seriously by all women who face the decision whether to take this elective medication or not.

In the United States deaths from cancer of the uterus have been declining for years largely due to early detection by the Pap smear. Over the past ten years the number of women taking estrogen replacement therapy has quadrupled. In the last four years cancer registries around the country have been reporting increases of up to 50 per cent in the incidence of cancer of the endometrium (lining of the uterus) in postmenopausal women. This increase is largely confined to affluent, white women over the age of 50, —the very women most likely to take ERT.

In December 1975 and January 1976 three studies were published in medical journals which, while they do not prove that exogenous (outside the body) estrogens cause cancer, strongly suggest that a cause and effect relationship exists between estrogen replacement therapy and cancer of the uterine lining. As a result the Food and Drug Administration is developing warning labels for ERT pills and a booklet for patients which will describe the risks a woman faces when using these drugs.

The new reports indicate that women who take ERT for a year or more are five to 14 times more likely to develop cancer of the uterus than women who don't take this drug. (*New York Times*, December 4, 1975). Dr. Kenneth J. Ryan of Boston Hospital for Women suggests that women who take ERT face a risk of cancer that is comparable to that of smoking one pack of cigarettes a day. The one-pack-a-day smoker raises her chance of death from lung cancer by 17 times. The risk of developing cancer from ERT can be put another way. One out of 1000 women per year who have not taken ERT and who have not had hysterectomies (surgical removal of the uterus) develop cancer of the lining of the uterus. For women who take ERT the rate rises to between one woman out of 125 to one woman out of 250. A study from a retirement community in Los Angeles found that among those women who took ERT the risk of developing cancer of the lining of the uterus was greater than their combined risk of developing cancer of the breast, lungs, ovary and colon (*New York Times,* December 17, 1975).

In January, 1976, *The New York Times* reported that an unpublished study indicated a relationship between ERT and the risk of breast cancer (Cerra, 1976). In August, *The Times* carried a piece on a new longitudinal study of nearly two thousand women who took estrogen drugs after menopause (Brody, 1976). This study showed that the use of estrogen was associated with 30 per cent more cases of breast cancer than anticipated. For those women who took ERT for 15 years, cancers developed twice as often as the expected rate.

Although until very recently it simply was not known whether exogenous (outside the body) estrogen is carcinogenic in human beings or not, there were clear indications that it might be. For instance it has been known for some years that large doses of estrogen given over a long period of time caused cancers in the following animals: mice, rats, rabbits, hamsters and dogs. These cancers developed in the breast, cervix, endometrium (lining of the uterus) pituitary, testicles, kidney and bone marrow (Seaman, 1975). It has also been known that estrogen encourages the growth of estrogen-dependent cancers, i.e. already existing cancers of the breast, ovaries or uterus. Removal of the ovaries has been used as a treatment for breast cancer because it often caused a remission of the disease.

In 1973 the Conference on Menopause and Aging reported that there is some evidence that *high* doses of estrogen may lead to changes in the endometrium (lining of the uterus) (Ryan and Gibson, 1973). These changes were recognized as a precancerous condition. *The Journal of the American Medical Association* reported on an article from *The Medical Letter on Drugs and Therapeutics* (JAMA, February 19, 1973). Under hazards of estrogen therapy were listed spotting, menorrhagia (excessive mentrual flow), nausea, breast tenderness, and fluid retention. Also, ERT "can increase the size of uterine fibroids (fibrous tumors), and *may be implicated in the development of malignant disease"* (p. 847) (emphasis added).

*The Medical Letter* advises against the routine prescribing of estrogen during and after the menopause because there is no adequate evidence that such treatment is beneficial and because exogenous estrogens *may promote or aggravate cancer of the genital organs or of the breast in some women.* (emphasis added).

Between 1945 and 1970 diethylstilbestrol (DES) was often given to pregnant women to prevent threatened miscarriage even though there was doubt about its efficacy and no statistical evidence to prove its value (Weiss, 1975). Weiss reports that 170 cases of cancer of the vagina have developed in the daughters of these women. After the first seven cases of this very rare disease appeared, one epidemiologist wrote that there appears to be a direct etiological (causal) relationship between DES taken by pregnant women and vaginal cancer in their female offspring. He compares it to other congenital effects which were caused by German measles or thalidomide therapy in the mother.

Cancer typically appears years after the original carcinogenic (cancer causing) stimulus. Every known human carcinogen, for example over-exposure to the sun, certain dyes, asbestos, vinyl chloride, nicotine, takes ten years or more to cause cancer. Then it may take another ten years before the cancer causes symptoms. This is why the relationship between estrogen in the Pill and cancer has been thought of facetiously by some medical professionals as "the time bomb with the 20-year fuse."

To conclude, a relationship between exogenous (outside the body) estrogens and cancer must now be assumed to exist. The millions of women taking ERT today are facing a substantially increased risk of developing cancer of the uterus or the breasts. The studies about ERT and cancer show that the longer estrogens are taken, the greater the risk of cancer. The dangers are clear.

It is not known what hazards, if any, the postmenopausal woman faces as a result of taking the birth control pill in her childbearing years. It is not known whether the fact that a woman took the Pill for a number of years has any effect on the cancer risks she faces if she takes ERT postmenopausally.

## 7. ESTROGEN REPLACEMENT THERAPY?

A panel of experts, obstetricians and gynecologists, who formed an advisory committee to the FDA, reported that there was a lack of valid scientific evidence to support the claims made for ERT. They suggested that the drug be used only for those conditions in which it is known to be effective. "But the panel was unable to determine these conditions" (Brody, 1975b, p. 38).

It is not thought likely that the FDA will ban Premarin, the drug which monopolizes the ERT market. Dr. Donald C. Smith who directed one of the studies in Seattle, Wash. says "This is an extremely valuable drug . . . but we will have to start using it more cautiously" (*New York Times*, December 4, 1975, p. 55). Dr. Harry K. Ziel of Los Angeles, director of the second study said about Premarin:

This is not an innocuous drug that can be used like salt and pepper. Doctors should restrict its use to women with incapacitating symptoms since it has a life-threatening risk (ibid).

He added that prolonged estrogen therapy was unjustified because the claims that it reverses aging and prevents bone loss are unproved.

## 8. ESTROGEN REPLACEMENT THERAPY— HOW LONG?

The FDA's advisory committee recommended that ERT should be used in the lowest dose and for the shortest time possible. They suggested it should be given on a stop and start basis, discontinuing it to check whether a woman needs it and to see if a lower dose is equally effective.

In 1973 the *Medical Letter* recommended short-term treatment with estrogen for vasomotor complaints (hot flashes and sweats) and atrophic vaginitis (thinning of the vaginal wall) (JAMA, Feb. 19, 1973).

Vasomotor disturbances ("flushing and sweats") may occur in some women, and may cause anxiety or depression; these patients could benefit from additional estrogen for several months to a year or two, after which therapy can be stopped (p. 847).

It was also stated that the estrogen replacement regimen is seldom indicated and involves some degree of risk.

The *AMA Drug Evaluations* (1974) recommends a woman should not take ERT therapy for more than two years.

## 9. ESTROGEN REPLACEMENT THERAPY— DOES IT POSTPONE SYMPTOMS?

Several of the women in the author's study reported that their hot flashes returned as soon as they went off estrogen medication. An older respondent wrote that her two sisters-in-law had been on estrogen in their 50's and 60's, but then developed mastitis (lumps in the breast). They were then taken off estrogen; now they are having hot flashes in their 70's. When one woman asked her gynecologist how long she would have to be on ERT, he told her about a patient in her 60's who stopped the pills, then began having hot flashes and returned to ERT. The implication that a woman might have to be on hormones for years and years started this individual questioning the treatment.

Several years ago, Dr. Isaac Starr (1974), retired professor of Research Therapeutics at the University of Pennsylvania, wrote the author:

The treatment for menopause is purely symptomatic. Though ERT is certainly effective in relieving symptoms, there is grave doubt that it doesn't merely postpone the end, i.e., symptoms return when you stop medicine and total amount is not much changed.

If you can get along without the temporary relief that the drugs bring, *do* so.

On the other hand, the drugs do relieve the symptoms and many patients are pleased by what they do, *so* most doctors give them, and certainly they do little if any harm.

(The statement that replacement estrogens are relatively harmless could not be made today.)

The question of whether menopause symptoms return when ERT is stopped is an important one. The author began ERT because of severe hot flashes. My gynecologist put me on the drug, increasing the dosage when the hot flashes returned, and from time to time took me off it "to see how I was doing." Each time I went off the drug, the hot flashes returned immediately. They seemed worse than ever. Under this program my body never had a chance to get permanently adjusted to the decreased amount of estrogen. I determined to stop the drug, live through the misery and get over the hot flash symptoms once and for all.

Two female physicians who believe in short-term ERT therapy both expect their patients to have some hot flashes when the dosage is reduced. A moderate female physician reported she could "wean" [sic] a woman off ERT after several years because by that time the hot flashes were less troublesome. A feminist M.D., who is sympathetic to women, reduces the dosage gradually until a woman is taking the lowest dose pill every other day. The regimen is flexible, however, so that if hot flashes are bad on a day without a pill, she suggests taking one and skipping the next day, or taking half a one. Several women in the author's menopause study corroborated the impression that the hot flashes that result from going off ERT are less intense than those which caused the women to take the drug originally.

The author knows of no study that has been done comparing the hot flash symptoms of the natural menopause with those that occur with withdrawal from ERT. One factor that could affect women's perceptions of the hot flashes resulting from going off ERT is that the women are now several years older and therefore may be less threatened by the notion of being menopausal women.

If it is true that taking ERT for several years merely postpones the symptoms of estrogen withdrawal, what has been gained by taking this drug? Before the new studies linking estrogens with cancer appeared, the author discussed this matter with a leading endocrinologist and asked him "What is the point of taking ERT for two years?" He replied, "No point at all." Nevertheless this endocrinologist believed that the advantages of long-term, low-risk individualized estrogen replacement therapy were worth the risks. When pressed for reasons for this position he mentioned that the main advantage of ERT is that *it breeds better health habits.* In other words, he felt ERT was worth taking because it brings a woman to the doctor every six months to have a physical checkup—this was the point he was making—and to have her prescription filled. The author asked him if a prescription-controlled placebo (dummy pill) wouldn't have the same advantages and no risks at all to the health of women.

## 10. THE TESTING OF NEW DRUGS

Fifteen years ago, Dr. Isaac Starr, Chairman of the Council on Drugs of the American Medical Association, wrote the lead article in the first annual *Therapeutic Number* of *The Journal.* The article was called "The Testing of New Drugs and Other Therapeutic Agents." He begins "Any doctor writing on methods of testing the effectiveness of new drugs and other therapeutic agents should do so with humility—for doctors have so often been mistaken about such matters" (1961, p. 2). He gave as an example of such errors Dr. Benjamin Rush's treatment of his patients by bloodletting and purging during the dreadful yellow fever epidemic in 1793. Rush was thought to be the hero of the epidemic. Years later he was accused of killing his patients by this treatment and he lost most of his practice.

Dr. Starr asked what happens when a new drug is developed? The physician is faced with a patient in distress. He wants to help, so he tries the new drug. If it appears to be beneficial, the doctor talks about it and later publishes it; if not, he tries something else and keeps quiet. Dr. Starr postulates a law: "For any new remedy, the favorable reports will appear before the unfavorable." Or, "Whenever a new remedy is introduced, there is likely to be a period when all the reports are favorable" (p.3). Isn't this exactly what has happened with ERT? Estrogen replacement seemed the perfect panacea. So the word went out. It is only after the passage of time and the recent longitudinal studies that the dangers and risks of taking this drug are being recognized and reported.

## 11. CONCLUSION

The facts about the physical side of the menopause have now been presented. Armed with the facts, each individual woman must balance the advantages as against the risks of medical therapy and decide how she wants to cope with this natural physiological change in her life.

**Comparison of medical and nonmedical therapies.** In an effort to help women with these decisions, Chart III presents medical and nonmedical therapies for the problems of menopause and aging, along with the advantages and risks of each. See pages 88-91.

The chart covers eight problems of menopause and aging. Only the first three are exclusively female problems.

**1. Hot flashes and sweats.** The problem of hot flashes and sweats and the advantages and risks of taking ERT for the small percentage of women who have these problems have been covered. Nonmedical therapy suggests accepting the discomforts of the climacteric because it is a natural, normal and healthy result of being a woman. Women can be glad to be rid of menstruation and worries about pregnancy and they can look foreward to feeling better, full of PMZ.

The end of menstruation, however, does not end the responsibility women have for preventive medical care of their bodies. They should continue with monthly breast examinations and with regular medical checkups, every six months to one year.

**2. Vaginal atrophy.** The percentage of women who suffer in later years from this problem is not reported in the literature so it is probably not known. ERT in pill form is effective although it would not be wise to take this strong drug for a purely local problem. ERT in cream form is also effective. This also poses some risk as the estrogen in the cream is absorbed through the walls of the vagina into the body system. The amount of risk is unknown.

The fear that they are going to "dry up" pushes some women into taking estrogens. Vaginal atrophy has been presented by medical authorities as the result of the decreasing supply of estrogen which occurs during the climacteric. However, the vagina, like any other muscle, will

88

# CHART III

## COMPARISON OF MEDICAL AND NONMEDICAL
## THERAPIES FOR PROBLEMS IN MENOPAUSE AND AGING

| Problem | Medical Therapy |
|---|---|
| 1. Hot flashes and sweats | ERT—under doctor's care, low dosage, short period of time |
| 2. Vaginal atrophy (painful intercourse) | ERT in pill form not recommended.<br><br>ERT in cream form for local application. |
| 3. Urinary stress, incontinence (involuntary urination with coughing, sneezing) | ERT in pill form not recommended.<br><br>ERT in cream form for local application. |
| 4. Osteoporosis (bone loss) (lower backache, fractures, dowager's hump) | ERT |
| 5. Heart attack | ERT |
| 6. Emotional problems | ERT |
| 7. Aging skin | Estrogen in skin cream |
| 8. Weight gain | |

| Advantages | Risks |
|---|---|
| Stops flashes and sweats. Regular every 6 months to a year physical exam including checkup of breasts, vagina, rectum, and Pap smear | Warning: may cause cancer of uterus or breasts.<br><br>Contraindicated for women with history of blood clots, or personal or family history of cancer; or for women with irregular bleeding or mastitis (non-cancerous tumors of breast).<br>Break-through bleeding may mask uterine cancer.<br>Some unpleasant side effects. |
| Stops vaginal atrophy. | Not recommended.<br>See above. |
| Stops vaginal atrophy. | Estrogen in cream will be absorbed into the system.<br>Amount of risks unknown. |
| Stops stress incontinence. | Not recommended.<br>See Vaginal Atrophy. |
| Stops stress incontinence. | Amount of risk unknown. |
| Not yet proven effective. | Questionable.<br>See above for risks. |
| Not effective in preventing heart attack | Not recommended.<br>May predispose to heart attack.<br>See above. |
| Not effective in emotional problems | Not recommended.<br>see above. |
| Not effective in preventing aging of skin | Not recommended.<br>See above. |

## CHART III

## COMPARISON OF MEDICAL AND NONMEDICAL
## THERAPIES FOR PROBLEMS IN MENOPAUSE AND AGING

| Problem | Nonmedical Therapy |
|---|---|
| 1. Hot flashes and sweats | Understand and accept the discomfort. It will pass in a year or two. Pay attention to total health care: physical, social, psychological. |
| 2. Vaginal atrophy (painful intercourse) | Regular sexual activity, self-sexual or otherwise. Exercise pubococcygeus muscle.<br><br>Use lubricating jelly. |
| 3. Urinary stress incontinence | Exercise pubococcygeus muscle. |
| 4. Osteoporosis (bone loss) (lower backache, fractures, dowager's hump) | Stress and strain of daily physical exercise. Good nutrition, especially enough calcium *and* vitamin D. Limit alcohol and certain anti-depressant drugs. |
| 5. Heart attack | Daily physical exercise. Stop smoking. Do not be overweight—diet: low in sugar and saturated fats, high in protein, raw vegetables, fruits, vitamins. |
| 6. Emotional problems | Feminist psychotherapy.<br><br>Join consciousness-raising group. |
| 7. Aging skin | Nothing will prevent aging skin, but keep out of the sun. Good nutrition. Moisturizers—a myth. Mineral oil for base; vaseline as night cream. Clean with Ivory or Neutrogena soap. |
| 8. Weight gain | Good nutrition. Fewer calories needed with age. Eat fruit, nuts, grains, vegetables and less animal fats. Regular physical exercise. |

| Advantages | Risks |
|---|---|
| No risks to health from taking strong female hormones. No side effects. PMZ: Postmenopausal zest. | Risk of not being responsible for regular physical checkup every six months to one year. |
| Sexual interest continues into old age. | None |
| May improve vaginal tone. Can improve sexual response. | None |
| Effective in improving mechanics of sex. | None |
| Effective in improving vaginal tone. | None |
| Physical fitness. | None |
| A healthy appearance. Look and feel well. | None |
| Enjoy living. | None |
| Physical fitness. | None |
| Will improve health. | None |
| Will improve health. Lower chance of heart attack. | None |
| Face problems of living. | Might make a woman face the real problems of her life. |
| Gain the support of other women. | Ditto |
| Too much sun is bad for the skin. | None |
| Healthy appearance. | None |
| Best preventive skin care. | None |
| Best cleansers. | None |
| Good physical health. | None |
| Less danger of heart attack. | None |

atrophy (waste away) from disuse. Dr. Ralph W. Gause (1970) remarks that the withdrawal of estrogen and the lack of sexual activity work together. "The estrogen level may fall but if the vagina is sexually active, it remains fully functional" (p. 65). He also believes that vaginal atrophy is reversible by giving estrogen or by resuming regular sexual activity.

Lack of use is one of the main causes for the decline of muscle tone in the body. Exercise is nothing more than regular physical activity. An active sex life, including sexual intercourse and/or masturbation is the best preventive for vaginal atrophy.

Non-medical therapy for vaginal atrophy suggests exercising the pubococcygeus or PC muscle, the muscle which runs from the pubic bone in front to the coccyx bone in the back. In it are the three female body openings. When a woman sits on the toilet with her legs far apart, then stops the flow of urine, she is using the pubococcygeus muscle. Women can learn to contract, to bear down and to hold the PC muscle. This exercise and others like it are known as "Kegels." Dr. Arthur Kegel developed a series of PC muscle exercises to help women with the common problem of urinary incontinence (Barbach, 1976, p. 52). The exercises have proved helpful to women in tightening the vagina after trauma from childbirth. They have also helped women learn to become orgasmic. They should prove helpful in conditions of vaginal atrophy.

In her book, *For Yourself*, Lonnie Barbach teaches Kegels to pre-orgasmic women. She writes that it is "quite important to keep this muscle, like others in your body, in tone. The exercises can become as much of a habit as brushing your teeth and, like brushing your teeth, they should be continued the rest of your life" (p. 56).

Various products can be used to help with a lack of lubrication. A lubricating jelly like K-Y Jelly can improve the mechanical side of sexual intercourse, it can be useful in masturbation and it has been successfully used by women to treat discomfort from dryness of the vagina. Oils can be helpful also. Try massage oil, baby, coconut or vegetable oil, but avoid oils with alcohol in them as they could irritate the genital mucus membranes (Barbach, 1976). Do not use a petroleum jelly like Vaseline because it isn't water soluble and if it gets in the vagina or urethra (canal to the bladder) it can cause problems.

**3. Urinary stress incontinence.** The frequency or rarity of this condition is unknown. Exercises of the pubococcygeus muscle have proved helpful.

**4. Osteoporosis.** The use of ERT for osteoporosis is of doubtful value to date. At a conference on the nutritional problems of women Dr. Louis V. Avioli commented on the normal bone loss experienced by women.

The reason for this age-related skeletal loss is still purely conjectural at best . . . Dietary indiscretion, inactivity, decrease in muscle mass, hormonal imbalance, renal dysfunction . . . have been implicated as causative factors.

Muscle mass seems very important to the integrity of bone . . . day to day muscle pulling through the tendons stimulates formation of bone (Nemy, 1975).

Muscle pulling is what you do when you exercise. Because one of the most commonly seen causes of osteoporosis is lack of physical activity, regular physical activity is important to counteract the normal bone loss in aging. Depending on an individual's age and physical condition, appropriate exercise would be walking, jogging, jumping rope, yoga class, exercise class, sports, etc.

Dr. Avioli suggested that certain drugs taken by depressed postmenopausal women cause mineral and protein to leech out of the bone (Nemy, 1975). Drinking alcohol also leads to bone loss according to this expert. Nonmedical therapies for preventing bone loss include regular exercise and avoiding alcohol and certain drugs.

**5. Heart attack.** ERT is not effective in preventing heart attack. An increased vulnerability to vascular accidents is clearly associated with taking estrogens.

Nonmedical therapies include daily physical exercise, not smoking, and controlling diet so as not to become overweight. Diet should be low in sugar and unsaturated fats, high in protein and high in raw vegetables, fruits and vitamins. Nonfadist books on nutrition, diet and vitamins are listed in the bibliography.

**6. Emotional problems.** ERT is not effective for emotional problems. Emotional problems in middle age appear to be due to the change in role that women are faced with when their children leave home, they are out of a job and they are looking foreward to growing old in America.

Therapy with a feminist psychotherapist may help a woman suffering from emotional pain. If the emotional problems are not severe, a consciousness-raising group can be helpful. The risks here are that therapy may help a woman confront the dissatisfactions in her life and thus recognize the relationship between her role as wife and mother and her pain. This might result in the rejection of these roles and the consequent loss of her livlihood.

Women should be aware that Valium, one of the most widely prescribed tranquillizers, is a depressant. It should not be taken if a person is feeling discouraged, hopeless and helpless.

**7. Aging skin.** There is no cure for aging skin. Neither ERT in creams, with the attendant risks, or expensive skin creams will stop the skin from aging. Since nothing ages the skin as fast as sunlight, keep out of the sun or, if in the summer sunlight, protect the skin with sun-screening lotions. Mineral oil can be used as a makeup base, and vaseline at night. Keep the skin clean with clear water and mild soap like Ivory or Neutrogena.

**8. Weight gain.** Gaining weight is not inevitable with aging. Because less calories are needed with age, the amount of calories consumed should be reduced. Regular physical exercise will help.

# Chapter 7_____

# WOMEN: MENOPAUSE AND MIDDLE AGE

*Women and Physical Health*

*Women and Social Health*

*Women and Psychological Health*

*Final Conclusion*

## 1. WOMEN AND PHYSICAL HEALTH

When women reach "the watershed age of 50" they are faced with many changes in their lives. Someone has said that living is problem solving; if you have no problems you might as well be dead. There are major problems for women to solve at this time in their lives and the solutions will not be easy. Even though new ways of living may come too late for this generation of women, they will make life easier for the women who follow.

The woman of 50 is not old. She is just beginning middle age. The years of maturity that lie ahead can be emotionally satisfying to her and a contribution to the society in which she lives.

## Preventive Health Care

**Women and physical health.** In order to take full advantage of the next 25 years, women must be in good health. Most middle-aged women are healthy. By practicing good preventive health care now, they can give themselves the best opportunity to remain that way. Women can learn new ways of thinking and feeling about their own bodies. Each woman needs to recognize that *she* is the person responsible for her body and for her own good health. It is an abnegation of personal responsibility to let medical people make decisions that affect one's body without investigating how the decisions are arrived at and reviewing the alternatives involved.

## Women and Doctors

Women need doctors. A middle-aged woman needs a well-trained responsible physician who is confident enough and flexible enough to provide the different kind of health care that women are beginning to demand today.

One major problem with the medical profession is that the right hand doesn't know what the left hand is doing. That is, the results of new studies or of conferences like the National Institute of Health one on Menopause and Aging (Ryan and Gibson, 1973) do not sift down to the busy doctor at the local level. It is particularly frightening to realize that most of the literature that the doctor gets about new drug products comes from the drug companies themselves. Their interest is primarily in profits and only secondarily are they concerned with the welfare of the people who take their medication.

Medical doctors do not know all the answers to the health problems of middle-aged women. When Dr. Forbes asked a symposium of medical people if it's good "to treat women for menopause?" (Ryan and Gibson, 1973, p. 270), he was implying that physicians themselves do not know whether menopause is a natural body development, a deficiency state or a disease process. Currently, doctors are taught very little about nutrition and are very poorly trained to deal with sexual problems. Moreover, physicians are limited according to their training. Thus, when surgeons are faced with medical problems, they think of cutting because that is their skill, and many unnecessary operations have been performed to the shame of the medical profession. For women this includes unnecessary hysterectomies (removal of the uterus), episiotomies (cutting the opening of the vagina to facilitate childbirth) and perhaps radical mastectomies (removal of the breast plus surrounding muscles and lymph nodes).

Fortunately, Americans are not as "sold on science" as they used to be. Feminists in particular have been pointing out the limitations in the health care establishment and its treatment of women.

Ninety-four per cent of obstetricians and gynecologists are male, and the figure for internists is about the same. (After a woman's reproductive life is over, there is no reason why she should continue with an obstetrician/gynecologist for her physician. A general practitioner or an internist may well be more appropriate because these doctors are concerned with a woman's total bodily health and not just the health of her reproductive organs.) The fact that most doctors are male introduces a further complication into women's learning to be responsible for their bodies. The socialization of women makes them overly respectful of male authority figures like doctors, psychiatrists, husbands and fathers.

**A new kind of woman-doctor relationship.** Women can develop a new relationship with their doctors. It will not be easy because the medical profession is conservative and is committed to maintaining the sex-role stereotypes of the past. Pauline Bart describes the image of women which is pictured in the OB-GYN textbooks. One textbook, 1971, reports: "The traits that compose the core of the female personality are feminine narcissism, masochism and passivity" (Huber, 1973, p. 286). Men who think of women this way, men who choose the obstetrical field because of special needs of their own, are not likely to respond comfortably to a woman who wants to learn how to be responsible for her own body.

Here is an example. One woman found she needed an increasing dosage of ERT to prevent the recurrence of hot flashes. When she told her gynecologist that she was thinking of going off the pills, his reply was a petulant "Well, you don't *have* to take them." The tone in his voice indicated that *his feelings* were hurt because his patient was rejecting his medication.

The new studies linking replacement estrogens with uterine and breast cancer will pose problems for women in relation to their physicians. Women will need doctors who will listen to their concerns, who will sensitively evaluate their symptoms when they have them, and who will describe the advantages and disadvantages of taking estrogen. Then they can decide what is the reasonable and responsible thing to do.

Some feminist women are going to their physician in pairs so one woman can give the other support while they work to put the doctor-female patient relationship on a new and more equal footing. One young woman was able to do this herself. She described her experiences as follows:

I went to my gynecologist yesterday for my annual checkup, dreading it as I do every year. However, I seriously doubt that I will feel that way again; I had a very good experience. I went there with the intention of talking to him about a few things, but more important, I went to his office with the conscious thought that it's my body and I have more of a right to know about it than he does.

When he took my blood pressure I asked him what it was. He mocked my question, asking me if it was a good one? I didn't mind terribly much as I felt strong inside and I knew that I was in the position of making this doctor-patient relationship more equal. A gynecologist can make these annual checkups demeaning—enough of that shit; nobody is going to make me ashamed of my body. I asked questions about anything I wanted to know about and commented on certain things. This examination was very different. I wasn't just a body on that table; he was dealing with me and my body.

After the examination we talked in his office. First thing I said was that it was long overdue that I call him by his first name. What does he like to be called? There was silence for a few seconds; he was very surprised. He made a quick recovery and when he remembered his name he told it to me. (The doctors and nurses call patients by their first names. I find it demeaning.) I made it a point to use it immediately—positive reinforcement. I was getting stronger and suddenly I loved it. Then I discussed Flagyl[1] with him and I told him that when he prescribed it for me and I asked him questions

---

[1] *Flagyl* is a drug used to treat trichomonas or "trich," the common vaginal infection. Eight studies have found it to cause cancer in rats and mice (Brody, 1975a).

about the possible side effects, I left his office with the distinct feeling that the thought it was not in my best interest to know about them. He minimized the importance of the side effects, but I wasn't to be deterred. I told him that I felt it necessary to get the answers to my questions and so I got an outside opinion. I told him that I don't ever want to have to get such satisfactions from another doctor again. We understood each other perfectly. I left his office, after discussing some other things, feeling strong and triumphant. I'll be damned if I'm ever going to allow anyone to treat my body as if it was a piece of machinery on an assembly line.

## Fashions in Medicine

Some years ago the feminist sociologist Pauline Bart (1968) wrote an aritcle called "Social Structure and Vocabularies of Discomfort: What Happened to Female Hysteria?" What she points out here is that there are what might be called fashions in illness that fluctuate with the attitudes current in that society. Thus female hysteria was prevalent among upper middle class women in Sigmund Freud's day whereas it is almost nonexistent today. Another medical fashion that was in vogue some 100 years ago was the practice of removing the ovaries. At that time it was thought that women's *psychology* was dominated by their reproductive organs. Thousands of ovariotomies were performed on women between 1860 and 1890 for *nonovarian conditions* (Ehrenreich and English, 1973). This major body cavity surgery was done when the mortality rate for such operations was far higher than it is today.

When the historical relationship between physicians and women is traced, it becomes possible to ask new questions about medical attitudes toward women today. Thus it is interesting to consider the swing in medical thought from the "natural ovariotomy" of not so long ago to today's ideas that the normal declining function of the ovary is a deficiency disease which requires continuous treatment with expensive medication made from female horses, medication which until recently had not been adequately tested.

A current medical fashion is the hysterectomy which is done on large numbers of women. Rogers (1975) reports that nearly half of all American women over 40 will be advised to have their wombs removed. *The New York Times* estimates that 787,000 hysterectomies were done during 1975 and 700 women died as a result. Twenty-two percent of these operations were not recommended and 374 women died unnecessarily (*New York Times*, Jan. 27, 1976). *The Times* suggests that many of the problems that this operation was supposed to solve could have been dealt with by more conservative and less dangerous methods. Rogers says that only ten to 20 percent of hysterectomies are caused by cancer or other life-threatening conditions. Studies have shown that the amount of surgery done in the USA is "directly related both to how many hospital beds and surgeons are available and the patients' ability to pay" (Rogers, 1975, p. 39).

In many cases of hysterectomy the woman's ovaries are also surgically removed although they show no pathology. The medical rationale for removing the ovaries is the danger of ovarian cancer later in life. Cancer of the ovary is not one of the leading cancers in women but it can be very serious when it occurs. The chance of this happening in a woman's 60's is about 100 to one. A reasonable decision here might be that a younger women should keep her ovaries if they are healthy, whereas a woman close to menopause might have them removed, especially if there was a family history of cancer. At any rate, *hysterectomies should not be done without getting a second medical opinion,* preferably from a physician who is not a surgeon, to be sure the operation is necessary at all.

### Selecting a Doctor

In selecting a physician for the middle years of life, a woman will be wise to find someone who will work cooperatively with her while they discuss together the climacteric and her own health care. She will need an M.D. who will take a full medical history to be sure no contraindications exist for the treatment they are considering. The physician should "individualize" any treatment suggested and not prescribe a lot of drugs in hopes something will do some good. If, together, a woman and her doctor feel that estrogen replacement therapy is wise for her, she will take a low dosage for a short period of time and only because the vasomotor symptoms of hot flashes and sweats are very disturbing indeed.

Regular medical checkups are important in middle life. These should include blood pressure, breast and rectal examination, an internal examination of the reproductive organs and a Pap smear. Medical opinion varies as to whether this should be done every six months or once a year. An office visit to a doctor costs money, as does the lab report on the Pap smear. In some places women are organizing Women's Health Services or clinics which will do these examinations at less cost.

Women can also do breast examinations on themselves once a month. Many women have a great reluctance to do this out of fear of what they may find. Women need to know that 65 to 80 percent of lumps in the breast turn out not to be malignant or cancerous. The earlier cancer is detected, the greater the chance of cure.

## Responsibility for One's Own Body

Women can develop a new attitude of responsibility for their bodies and for their own good health which goes beyond learning about menopause and choosing a new kind of medical doctor. It means paying attention to their total health care. Many factors determine physical health and length of life. Women cannot control their heredity or the quality of the air they breathe but they can do something about the food they eat, the amount of physical activity they get and about smoking cigarettes.

## Proper Nutrition

American diets are too high in fats and sugars. "Such diets can be contributing factors to obesity, heart and circulatory diseases, and diabetes" says the 1975 Yearbook of the U.S. Department of Agriculture (*Nutrition Action,* January 1976, p.2). It is recognized that overweight contributes to many physical disorders. Life insurance data suggests that people who are at their appropriate body weight have lower blood pressure, less heart disease and less cancer. There appears to be a negative relationship between the intake of dietary fat and life expectancy. The higher the amount of fat, the shorter the life span. What causes this is not known. It does need to be studied because the trend throughout the world is for people to introduce more fats into their diets (Schlenker *et al,* 1973).

Putting on weight is not inevitable in middle age. Becoming fat and dowdy is not a consequence of the climacteric but is a function of not reducing the intake of calories at a time when many people become more sedentary. It is also a result of no longer caring about one's physical appearance.

A balanced diet is still the best way to get an adequate supply of vitamins. Vitamins have become a food fad lately and many people are spending a lot of money on vitamin products. Dr. Roslyn Alfin-Slater, a professor of nutrition, says "It's a myth that depleted soil requires this" (*New York Times,* Nemy, 1975). Do not overdose with vitamins, especially vitamins A and D. Vitamin E is considered a magic pill today. In general, less than 300 International Units daily will not cause problems.

The natural foods movement is a reaction to the kind of food produced for Americans by an agribusiness which is more interested in profits than in nutrition. The natural foods movement makes some good points about the dangers of pesticides, chemicals and additives in the food we eat, about the need for whole grains instead of refined flours and about avoiding refined sugar, junk food and foods with "empty calories." However the difference between natural, or organic, and unnatural products is not as clear as it is made out to be. Many of their products are overpriced and no better for your health than the supermarket variety. Margolius' book, *Health Foods; Facts and Fakes,* (1973) makes good sense out of the conflicting claims coming from the health food movement.

If you are concerned about the chemical additives in food, you can avoid beef which still has DES added to it, stay away from sodium nitrites in bacon and other cured meats, and avoid red food coloring. One solution is to grow your own vegetables and freeze enough for the winter. A vegetable garden gives many benefits beyond the nutritional ones. It requires physical labor and growing things is good for the soul.

Clearly the best preparation for a healthy middle and old

age is a lifetime of good diet. Unfortunately, few Americans have been concerned with good nutrition and not a great deal is known about nutrition in the later years. (The especial nutritional needs of pregnant and lactating women have been the subject of much research.)

In an article on "Nutrition and Health of Older People" the authors state:

Proper nutrition throughout life has been suggested as one of the best means of minimizing the degenerative changes and their superimposed diseases. The dilemma is a specification of proper nutrition. There is, in fact, little useful evidence on which to base this specification (Schlenker et al, 1973, p. 1111).

Studies of three communities around the world where the inhabitants live to a very great age show that in all of them the people have meager low-caloric diets. The food consumed is not only low-calorie but it is also low in animal fats and proteins. The people eat mostly vegetables, rough grains and fruit (Cherry and Cherry, 1974). Columbia University's Institute of Human  Nutrition hosted a conference on the special nutritional demands of women. At it Dr. Avioli suggested that after the age of 30, women should watch their diets more carefully. He recommended protein as a necessary substance, not just animal protein, and he wondered if we should all be vegetarians (*New York Times*, Nov. 22, 1975).

Americans have been sold on the notion that good nutrition and high protein are synonymous (Machta and Jacobson, 1976). Reasonable amounts of protein are essential to good health but Americans eat about twice the recommended amounts and many people eat 3 and 4 times the RDA (recommended dietary allowance). Adequate protein can be obtained without eating meat by serving complimentary forms of vegetable protein. Frances Moore Lappé's book, *Diet for a Small Planet* (1971), shows how this can be done.

Bone loss appears to be a normal part of aging. A balanced diet, adequate amounts of calcium and vitamin D which is necessary for the absorption of calcium from the small intestine, and regular physical exercise may retard this condition.

**Exercise.** "Exercise is the closest thing to an antiaging pill now available," reports a specialist in human aging (Cherry and Cherry, 1974, p. 84). There are no rocking chairs or park benches in the communities where the people live so extraordinarily long. "Even the old men and old women purported to be 130 are supposed to work at least a few hours each day" (p. 82). Women need to exercise regularly to keep their bodies fit. One of the best preventive measures a person can take against both heart attack and osteoporosis (bone loss) is regular physical activity.

**No smoking.** Smoking should be avoided. The rate of heart attack in women has risen in direct relation to the increase in women's smoking. The death rate for cancer of the lung in women has doubled in the past ten years. Lung cancer is now the third leading cause of cancer in women. Women's deaths from lung cancer used to be one-sixth the death rate of men. Today it is one-fourth and catching up (*Cancer Facts and Figures,* 1975). For a feminist, it is most distressing to read that there has been a substantial increase in smoking among teen-age girls in the past six years. Women who care about their bodies will not smoke cigarettes.

**Sexual health.** The responsible use of a woman's sexuality is no less important in middle age than it was when a woman was younger. A good rule is, no more sex than you are ready for. How a woman uses herself sexually relates directly to her feelings about herself as a person. Your body is you. Psychological health is just as important as physical health.

Although pregnancy is no longer a problem in middle age (you can expect not to get pregnant if you have not had a period for at least one year), venereal disease is prevalent. You should familiarize yourself with the symptoms of the diseases that it is possible to get from close physical contact. Not only syphilis and gonorrhea but also herpes-2, venereal warts, and the parasites crabs or pubic lice and scabies or mites.

If you are sexually active, a regular gonorrhea test is recommended. If two people in a relationship, heterosexual or homosexual, start out the relationship "clean," and they are monogamous, that is, they do not have sexual relations with other partners, this would not be necessary.

**Preventive health care.** In an article, "Our Goal is Health not Medical Care," Herman M. Somers (1975), makes the point that the greatest potential for improving the health of the American people will not be found in training more doctors or in building more hospitals "but rather in what people can be taught and motivated to do for themselves, in influencing personal behavior and attitudes" (p. 13). He quotes a medical historian who 35 years ago warned that we may be in danger of becoming an over-medicated society and exposing ourselves more and more to iatrogenic (drug-induced) illness. He concludes with a quotation, "The state can protect our society very effectively against a great many dangers, but the cultivation of health, which requires a definite mode of living, remains to a large extent, an individual matter" (*ibid*).

## 2. WOMEN AND SOCIAL HEALTH

The way a woman is integrated into her society can be viewed as a measure of her social health. In this society women are socialized to become wives and mothers. While they are in the child-rearing stage of the family life cycle, many women feel comfortable and happy with what they are doing, thus reflecting the views of the society around them that they are behaving appropriately. There are of course many real satisfactions in the child-rearing and housekeeping tasks, which is why women have accepted and even enjoyed these roles and not complained about their second-rate status. However, when the children leave home, if a women isn't already employed for pay or doesn't have to seek such work, "the woman is often placed in a 'social vacuum,' and this is not always compensated for by cultural and political activities" (van Keep and Kellerhals, 1973, p. 162). This quotation about the problems of middle-aged women comes from an article on "The Aging Woman" written in Switzerland. The problem of older women is endemic in Western society.

### The Need to Find a New Role

The accepted social role for a married woman today includes three areas: wife, mother and housewife. In middle age some women lose the wife role, mothering is ended or will be shortly and only the housewife role is left. A major problem then facing middle-aged women who have lived the traditional home, husband and child-centered life is to find a new central role or occupation for themselves. Society has not prepared women for this discontinuity in their lives.

**Women and housework.** A discussion of women and their relationship to housework is a complicated one. As every woman knows, housework is as much real work as any work that is done for pay. Oakley (1974b) has broken down the job of housework into six basic activities: cleaning, shopping, cooking, washing up (doing the dishes), washing clothes and ironing. Ironing has about disappeared from the American scene but Vanek (1974) suggests that more time now is being spent in family management than used to be the case. In Oakley's study of 40 English housewives, nearly half reported that the best thing about being a housewife is that you are your own boss; and the worst thing is the housework itself with its monotony, repetitiveness and boredom. Housework is a never ending job. Another disliked aspect of housework is the social isolation. Not surprisingly, one of the most liked of the six basic household activities is shopping. Among the housewives studied by Oakley, shopping tended to be a daily activity.

Betty Friedan pointed out many years ago that housework expands to fill the time available. Oakley calls this "job enlargement." It is quite clear that unless a woman is a "houseproud housewife," that is a woman who is psychologically very heavily invested in her housekeeping chores, there is no reason why housework needs to take so many hours. Vanek's study of housework found that non-employed women spent nearly twice the time on housework as did employed women even though other factors like the number of children were kept constant. Moreover she found that non-employed housewives spent more time in housework chores on evenings and weekends than did employed women. She explains this puzzling finding by suggesting that because the value or the worth of their housework is not clear to women—that is, women feel they are not contributing as much to the family as their husbands who earn wages—they make themselves spend long hours at it. "Non-employed women schedule work so that it is visible to others as well as to themselves" (p. 120).

Why are women so tied into the housewife role? They are able autonomously to determine the standards that will prevail in their houses as to neatness, cleanliness, cooking etc. and they are able to set up their own schedules for doing this work. In discussing this issue, Oakley makes the very good point that women in developing their notions of the feminine role have learned the lessons of childhood too well. Women have served a long apprenticeship learning the female role. A little girl plays house and rehearses the housework tasks. She imitates her mother and when she marries she repeats her mother's household behavior which she now thinks of as her own. The result is that housework becomes the feminine responsibility. Oakley concludes that "A fundamental challenge to the traditional equation between feminity and domesticity is hardly possible so long as the roots of domesticity remain firmly embedded in female personality and self-image" (p. 133).

Of course all the TV and magazine advertising aimed at selling household products to women hooks right into this feminine over-identification with housework.

So, knowing no other way to be feminine, women continue in the housewife role into middle age. Even though less and less housework *needs* to be done because of automation, convenience foods, better housing conditions, etc. (Oakley, 1974b) and because of the departure of the children, women continue to work long hours at it. There is great social waste of women here.

**No financial security in being a housewife.** Unless their husbands are well off or they have money of their own, there is no financial security for housewives. People in the paid work force are the best protected people in our society today. But the non-employed, especially housewives, are left at risk. Because they haven't worked for pay they get no health, retirement or unemployment benefits. They get no paid vacation time and their social security benefits, which they cannot get in most cases until they are 60 years old, are minimal. Homemakers, because their work is not considered "work," fall through the chinks of the social system. This problem is very well described by Cynthia Gorney (1976) in "The Discarding of Mrs. Hill".

108

**Middle-aged women alone.** Today there are many middle-aged women alone. Some are widows. Laurie Shields of the Alliance for Displaced Homemakers reports that there are 12 million widows in the USA with an average age of 56. An increasing number of middle-aged women are divorced. In many cases the new no-fault divorce law has meant increased financial hardship for women because support payments for women are lower and often are set for a limited period of time.

### Finding a Job

For a woman trained only in nurturing and housekeeping activities, the kind of job available, if one can be found, will not be likely to offer satisfaction in the areas of skill, status or financial rewards. Such a woman who tries to find a job at 40-50 has three strikes against her: her age, her sex, and her lack of relevant skills. The Davidoff and Markewich (1961) study found that the women who were able to find good jobs for themselves after the children were grown were women who had fitted paid jobs into their lives while they were mothers. Their careers were in the usual feminine occupations of nurse, teacher, social worker and librarian. Among the sample of 50 college-educated women studied, only four were in paid employment full-time and ten part-time.

Women's status relative to men's has declined in the past 25 years. Women consistently get paid only three-fifths of what men get paid for the same work. In the 45-to-50-year-old bracket, women earn only 54 percent of what men the same age are earning. "These discrepancies are due in large part to the kind of jobs women hold. They reflect the difficulties faced by mature women when they enter the labor force or reenter it after a period of absence" (*New York Times,* Sept. 15, 1973, report from a Conference on Aging).

This is the situation described in "The Discarding of Mrs. Hill" (Gorney, 1976). Mrs. Hill was a 53 year old widow who had to go to work after her husband died. The only work she could find was part-time in a nursing home. Today there are not enough jobs for all the people who want them so older women, teenagers and black people are unable to find work.

The lack of opportunity to work creates severe problems for women who need paid employment in order to survive.

**A Maternal Bill of Rights.** Alice H. Cook suggests a maternal bill of rights for women. She takes the GI Bill as an example of how the country repaid its returning soldiers for the years that they contributed to the defense of their country. They had interrupted their work lives for this task, losing their earnings and the training in job skills they would have had. Cook compares the years the GIs gave up to the years that women lose when they leave the labor force to have children "incidently a service to society incomparably more necessary and useful than the sacrifices war demands of men"(Cook, 1975, p. 67). Such a program would allow women to work part-time while their children are young, it would provide counseling and guidance, it would offer retraining or new training, and it would assist women with their reentry into the labor market.

These ideas are visionary, but they are a real goal to work toward.

**Conclusions about women and jobs.** The facts are that the opportunities for women of middle age to find suitable work are very small indeed. Shields says these women have the highest rate of unemployment of any section of the work force. But they can't get unemployment insurance because they worked at home and never worked in the paid labor force. They are ineligible for Social Security benefits because they are too young. They're ineligible for welfare unless they have dependent children, unless their grown children are unable to support them, unless they have no other income and their housing costs are less than $96.00 per month. Yet they are every bit as unemployed as an unemployed factory worker.

**Programs in other countries.** Cook (1975) reports that many countries, for example Germany, Australia, Austria, and Israel, have set up special offices and orientation programs for women who want to return to work. Sweden is the only Western nation with training programs for mature women and a policy of opening up new occupations for them that are outside the traditional women's job areas.

Sweden regards reentry into the work force as a decisive moment in a woman's life, a point at which with good planning and a little effort she can be made aware of the fact that she has a long work life ahead, that she will probably work during most of it, that investment in even brief training or in completion of schooling can pay off significantly not only in income but in job satisfaction, and that a new start at this juncture could include consideration of a start in a new occupation (Cook, 1975, p. 45).

**Programs in the United States.** The United States government is doing very little about this problem. Women are not placed very high on the national list of priorities. Women have been relatively powerless in American society so that their grievances are not well known.

NOW's Task Force on Older Women is working in coalition with the Alliance for Displaced Homemakers (ADH) to try and find some solution to this problem. California is the first state to have passed a Displaced Homemakers Bill. The aim is to get national legislation. A Displaced Homemakers Center is in the process of being established with funds from the state of California. The Center's goal is to maximize the chances for older women to get jobs. The Center expects to provide job training and on-the-job experience. They will try to create new jobs for women, they will encourage self-employment and they will develop full and part-time jobs.

There's a group called Washington Opportunities for Women (WOW) which has been pioneering for the past ten years in this field (Clevenger, 1975). In 1972 the U.S. Department of Labor's Manpower Administration provided funds to them to help set up similar self-help groups in six other communities: Atlanta, Richmond, Baltimore, Providence, Boston and White River Junction, Vermont. WOW does counseling, career guidance, and a program in high schools called "Careers for Peers." They have run four on-the-job training programs for low income women which had guaranteed well-paying jobs waiting at completion. They are doing a pilot program in work-rehabilitation for women probationers which provides secure employment for them. The staff at WOW has been working toward developing new jobs for women in non-traditional fields. They have been successful in training women for jobs in construction skills and in operating sewage treatment plants.

These two examples of women organizing programs to help other women find jobs are exciting and encouraging. The women who developed these programs at first were volunteers. They learned many of their organizational and management skills in volunteer work.

## Women and Volunteer Work

If a woman does not have to work for a living, volunteer work can be worth doing. Volunteer work comes in great variety, some of it is valuable and worthwhile, and it is not necessarily menial and unskilled work. There is a trend towards professionalizing volunteer work and more and more volunteer programs are requiring training of volunteers and a commitment to a certain number of hours a week to the volunteer job. In England, the National Marriage Guidance Council is a voluntary agency entirely staffed at the counselor level by volunteers. These people, men and women, are rigorously selected, then trained in marriage counseling skills and finally well-supervised for a certain amount of time. They are required to give a specific number of hours a week to their marriage counseling duties.

In volunteer work a woman has far more choice about the kind of work she'll do than she'd have in looking for a paid job. The kind of volunteer job selected should tie in with the goals that a woman sets for herself in what she wants to do with the rest of her life. Volunteer work can offer a woman the chance to grow personally, to develop new skills and to assume some responsibility. Moreover, when it is Valid Volunteering, to use Tish Somers' phrase, it can have real social impact. Let me suggest that women in America need all the help they can get.

## Advice for the Future

For the future, though, we can tell our daughters to prepare for the middle years of their lives while they are still young. Marriage and child-rearing are no longer an adult career for women. A woman must have a larger focus, a career field, an area of creative interest, a commitment to some "work." After they get some training or skills, we can tell them, they can expect to work in this field for a number of years until they drop out of it for childbearing and child-rearing. If they have chosen wisely, they will be able to work part-time at their "work" while the children are growing up. Later, when the children are older or have left home, a woman can return to her "work" full time.

Before the prospects for women and women's work change very markedly, two things must happen. The first is that society must change and there must be a broadening of opportunity for jobs for women. Both the government and business need to learn new and practicable ways to employ them (Clevenger, 1975). Secondly, women must change. It may be too late for some women whose lives are already set, but other women must begin to change their notions of what life will be like for them.

## Women Must Work Together

The author is not at all sanguine that the changes needed in our social system relevant to women and the paid labor force will be forthcoming in the near future. In fact, whenever the country moves into a severe depression, the number of paid jobs available for women decreases and the small gains that women have made toward equal employment are lost. Nevertheless, women must work together to continue to exert pressure for social change. The Women's Political Caucus is one of the most hopeful signs in this direction. Women must use their political power to be sure they are represented where the real decisions are made so that the needs of women can be adequately met.

At the very minimum, women need to be able to live in some kind of comfortable relationship with the society around them. At best women should be able to feel that they have been and will be, as long as they are able, active and productive and important members—not second class citizens—of their own society. The Women's Liberation Movement is the most significant social force working for women today. To make this society a better place for women is a tremendous job which can be done when women organize for political power.

## 3. WOMEN AND PSYCHOLOGICAL HEALTH

What do women worry about? They worry about the fact that every single day, they are getting older and less attractive. They don't worry about it consciously, or continually, but they do worry about it unconsciously, because there's not much a woman has to sell, in our society, except the way she looks.

What happens to a bright young woman in this society? She grows up and she gets married . . . She is a wonderful wife and mother . . . She does all the things she is supposed to do . . . She gets to the watershed age of 50 . . . a catastrophe has occurred . . . the kids have grown up. She has given them her life and they want only their own lives . . . She is menopausal. When she was young, she had raging hormones, and who wanted her in a tough job of top responsibility with raging hormones? Then her hormones stop raging and she is a menopausal woman. Who wants a menopausal woman around?

(Estelle Ramey, "She Is Woman," *New York Times,*
*Sept. 24, 1973, p. 33)*

It is tough to be a woman in America today, especially an older woman. The amount of emotional malaise among women is testament to this fact. Twice as many women as men are treated with psychoactive drugs for the various symptoms of frustration and unhappiness. Gornick and Moran (1971) discuss how women are taught that there is nothing so unpleasant, unworthy, and unattractive as an unhappy woman so they try to keep their miseries to themselves.

But women are learning that the dissatisfactions of each individual woman are really common to many women because they are a reflection of "woman's place" in this society. Women are learning that the attempt to adjust women to fit the traditional sex roles is emotionally damaging to them. What needs to be changed is the society and the sex roles themselves so that both women and men have equal opportunities for self-development.

### Finding Out Who You Are

One of the main tasks of middle age, and one of the most difficult, is to develop a new conception of the self. In order to cope well with this time in her life, a woman should give up being primarily "mother" or "wife" and become an independent person (though still a mother and sometimes still a wife). The proper time for developing a sense of identity is considered by psychologists to be late adolescence and early adulthood. It is an anomaly of our culture that so many women have to do this in middle age. Gloria Steinem uses the term "man junkies" to describe the female dependency on males that our society fosters.

**Leaning on men.** Sonya O'Sullivan (1975) describes beautifully this dependency and the outgrowing of it in "Single Life in a Double Bed." The article describes the feelings of a wife of 30 years as she goes from learning about her husband's mistress, through the divorce, the pain of separation and the pain of recovery.

On no fixed day, Mrs. is aware that she is suffused with a large inner smile. Of course, lacking sensuality, it is not a celebration. There is an absence of tambourines and castanets. She is at peace with her bitter freedom, and more. It is as though she were standing up straight for the first time. She understands that she was always leaning, so that, when Mr. moved away from her side, she fell. She knows, too, that she will fall again—and get up again. There is nothing easy about it. Just because of that, the pleasure is profound . . . Whatever she does, there will always be the deep pride of the survivor. (p. 52)

**Marriage is not an occupation.** O'Sullivan has Mrs.'s daughter write to her. "Frankly, I never did understand what you were doing with your life. Marriage is not an occupation. It is a personal arrangement. Now you're free to be you" (*ibid*). Yes, but who am I? wonders Mrs.

Gorney (1976) describes how 20-30 years ago women made a contract with their husbands: I'll stay home and you support me. However according to the March 1974 census, 37 percent of women over 40 have no husbands. Child-rearing women have finished that work after 20 years and they have 25 more years of life ahead of them. These women must find some other commitment in their lives, some other work.

**Your mission as a person.** The psychologist Robert Strom (1975) discusses work in "Education for a Leisure Society." Although his article is about how men in a leisure society need to change their notions about jobs and work, his concepts apply equally well to women and the problems facing them today. Strom makes a clear distinction between a person's work and a job or employment. He describes work as "your mission as a person, the activity you pursue with a sense of duty and from which you derive a self-meaning and a sense of personal worth" (p. 94). He goes on to say that our society is slowly realizing that

. . . what is important is not that each of us holds a job but that all of us have work. Many people who have jobs lack work and therefore a sense of satisfaction and self-pride. The problem cannot be solved just by making jobs more meaningful because there is a significant difference between having a work and holding a job. Nothing framed in a period shorter than a lifetime can be termed a man's work, but he may never have a job or may retire at age 60. (p. 95)

This author wouldn't agree that one's work has to be a lifetime association because people grow and mature and have different commitments, or work, at different times in their lives. In Strom's terms though, the woman in middle age needs to determine what her mission as a person will be from then on. This work is separate from a job, paid work or housework, that she does. Thus Mrs. Hill will have to work part-time in a menial job in a local nursing home because this is the only job she can get and she has to have the income. But her work might be the effort she puts into getting laws passed to give social security benefits to women who have spent 30 years doing housework. Another woman's job might be being a housewife and companion to her husband. But her work would be setting up or working at a good child-care facility for the children of working mothers. Or working at a Center for Displaced Homemakers helping other women get on their feet financially and emotionally.

**Make the choice early.** This notion of work as an important choice for woman should be pushed back in time. It is a choice that ought to be made, for women and men in early adulthood. If this were done then, housework could never become work—as it has for so many women in the past—but would be recognized as a job that is part of the necessary business of life. Home would be a place where food, clothing, cleanliness, privacy and intimacy are obtained by all the members of the family. Seen this way housework is something to be shared by husbands and children in line with their abilities. Reasonable standards would be set up according to the family's preferences. For instance, each could do his/her own laundry, and the housework would be done as expeditiously as possible.

**A mid-course correction.** Women in middle age have the chance to make what the Hunts (1975) call a "mid-course correction". A time to change the direction of one's life. If this hasn't been accomplished before, there is a chance now to search for some work, in Strom's sense, that will have a social, creative, moral or intellectual purpose and out of which a person can gain some sense of achievement and recognition. Such work should have the opportunity for personal growth and it must be intrinsically rewarding. Suzanne Keller has written in "Ethics for the Future" that in the future "A part of everyone's stay on earth can then be spent doing something he (she) enjoys, is good at, or is needed for" (Keller, 1970, p. 11).

**Who am I?** Before a woman can determine the direction of her life she needs to get in touch with herself and find out who she is.

There is a 'me' who isn't somebody's anybody, hidden beneath all the encumbrances natural to a woman's life. It is a 'me' who must choose what I could, would or should do with my twenty extra years (Reed and Phaltz, 1974, p. 18).

It may take a while to get to know yourself, to feel good and freindly about yourself, but it is a task worth doing. Some women do it by themselves, others do it in consciousness-raising groups, others in therapy.

Vicarious living is really not satisfactory. Women must learn to take their satisfactions from their own achievements. Two Junior League women wrote a book called *Stop the World, We Want to Get On* (Reed and Pfaltz, 1974). The title indicates the need that women are feeling, and expressing today, to have an effect on the real world outside their homes. The authors write

There is no prepared script for becoming a person . . . We need to feel the impact of our own individuality. We want personally to experience a proof of contact with life—a sense of having an effect . . more than our husband's position and our children's accomplishments (p. 18).

**Tell our daughters.** Unfortuantely many young women are still thinking that the real satisfactions of life will come from marriage and children. They haven't caught up with the fact that in today's world child-rearing, and often marriage too, is a temporary job. They don't appreciate that on the average they will spend 43 years in paid employment so it is important that it be work they like and want to do.

Because of the Women's Liberation Movement many young women believe they can combine the careers of mothering and work. They do not understand the burden of childrearing as it is institutionalized in our society and the very real limits it puts on achieving in the work world.

They have no idea of the time it takes to care for a young child. The child development textbooks say that the infant sleeps 80 percent of the time so why can't they go to graduate school, finish an article, put that new glaze on a pot while s/he is sleeping? Young women do not know that it is terribly expensive to employ a good person to care for a child, if one can be found; they do not realize that there are only 900,000 places for children in day care and there are six million children who need those places already. The quality of the day care available is another matter. Such unreal expectations as to what life is like will make for even more emotional dissatisfactions for our daughters than their mothers' generation experienced.

There is no easy solution and certainly no immediate solution to these conflicts. We can at least tell young women it is not all as easy as it seems. Unfortunately they will have to find out for themselves.

## 4. FINAL CONCLUSION

This book began with a discussion of the climacteric and menopause, so it is fitting that it should end on the same subject. The physical side of the change of life is not the real difficulty for women; it is the society that women live in.

Psychologically the end of reproduction should not be a great loss for women who have different attitudes towards fertility than in the past and who have voluntarily limited their reproduction for the previous 20 years.

## Women are Different From Men

Due to both nature and nurture, women are physically and emotionally different from men. These differences should not carry with them any implication of difference in inherent value or worth, but the fact is—painful though it may be to accept—that women are systematically treated as though they were of less value.

However this may be, to be a woman involves great pleasures and great joys. It can also involve a lot of bodily discomforts which are not indicative of illness or disease. Most women have experienced pain with menstruation at some time in their lives. There are discomforts during the first and last trimesters of pregnancy. Childbirth involves much stretching of the cervix, vagina and perineum (area between the openings of elimination), much of which is distressing and some of which is painful. Lactation can be uncomfortable. The climacteric and menopause can cause physical discomfort also.

Aches and pains are a part of living. Anyone who develops, trains and uses the body—a dancer, an athlete—knows and accepts this fact. If women understood more about their bodies and if they felt more proud and more responsible for them, they would not need to run to doctors for pills to eliminate every physical and mental ache and pain.

## Talk About Menopause

There is a strong taboo about talking about menopause, but women should talk to other women about this process all women have to go through. Young girls talk to each other about beginning menstruation, and this talking together helps them accept it psychologically. But most women do not talk about the climacteric with other women, (or even with their husbands), so they are deprived of the support other women could give them.

Women talking to women could dispel the myths about menopause. Menopause wouldn't be so frightening if women talked about its advantages in phsycial and emotional health and the PMZ (postmenopausal zest) they have to look forward to.

Women could learn about each other's physical complaints and they could help each other to master the temporary discomforts of this transition period. For instance, some women with severe flashes find that a complete yoga breath, as a hot flash begins, is helpful. Hot flashes and sweats are less uncomfortable if cotton clothing rather than synthetic is worn. If hot flashes are troublesome, take a skiing vacation in a cold climate rather than a swimming vacation in a hot one. Today people can learn to turn off migraine headaches; why can't women learn to turn off hot flashes?

Middle age consciousness-raising groups could help women deal with the prejudices this society has against women over 30. Women could encourage each other to develop themselves and find new interests and skills. A feminist photographer, the young woman who took my photograph, said that it was her consciousness-raising group which encouraged her to begin her career in photography.

Women talking, caring and sharing can help each other.

## Menopause, One of the Natural Processes of Life

One of the major life experiences of women is childbirth. There is a movement which is attempting to humanize this experience by encouraging and teaching women to give birth at home. This movement is founded on certain principles which can apply very well to women during the climacteric.

The following quotation was found in the afterward of a book on home birth.

We have to have faith in the life processes. Doctors in general have lost faith. Technical skill, though it may enhance faith can never supplant it, and many doctors are no longer able to distinguish health, as epitomized by [menopause][1] from illness (Brown, 1972, no page).

---

[1]This author substituted "menopause" for "pregnancy".

Doctors who assist at home births have found what appears to be a remarkably lower incidence of postdelivery "blues" than is found in hospital deliveries (Lang, 1972). Surely if the climacteric were attended by other women in the same way that home birth is, the number and severity of complaints and symptoms would also be reduced. Women can learn to trust the naturally unfolding processes of their lives. The climacteric is one of these. Women together can "tend and heal and share each other's growth".

The climacteric and menopause are the ending of one phase of life and the beginning of another. Menopause is not a disease. It is an opportunity for growth.

# Appendix 1

# PILOT STUDY ON MENOPAUSE

My menopause study was an exploratory one. I wanted to discover from women directly what they had experienced or what they were presently experiencing from the climacteric. I talked about menopause with as many menopausal or post-menopausal women as I could find. The discussions which I led after giving a talk on menopause became an excellent place for this kind of information sharing. I advertised in *The Monthly Extract*, *Alert* and *Prime Time* stating that I was writing a position paper on menopause for the National Organization for Women's Task Force on Older Women and asking for documentation of individual experiences. In addition, I wrote to individuals and to groups of women working on the subject seeking access to any information they had compiled.

Information gathered in this manner cannot be considered statistically significant. Furthermore, it cannot be generalized to all women. But, it is at least a beginning, and I think a good one, towards finding out from women themselves just what the climacteric really was/is for them.

The second part of my study took the form of a short questionnaire which I passed out at my 30th college reunion. I asked permission from the Chairone to distribute the anonymous questionnaire at the close of the first meeting of the class. She agreed, but when the time came, it was forgotten. When I stood to remind her, she introduced me and commented on the project, but with gratuitous remarks to the effect that I was going to suggest that "we give up Premarin." Her remarks were brief, but the incident illustrates the deep feelings many women have about menopause and about how important their ERT pills are to them. Despite the pejorative introduction, about half the women present, or 28 filled in the questionnaire. The questionnaire is discussed on pages 64, 66.)

Some of the questions I asked were: Do you have hot flashes? How long have you been having them? Have you noticed a change in their nature? How troubling are they? Can you turn them off in any way?

# Appendix 2

# THREE EXERCISES

Following my Menopause and Middle Age workshops, the participants and I do three pencil and paper exercises. These exercises have proved to be helpful. The process of translating your life from the memories in your mind into a diagram on paper often brings new understanding and new perspectives. Some women find the exercise results in increased confidence about their middle and older years. My own experience agrees.

## EXERCISE 1

### Draw Your Own Life-line

Your life-line is an actual line which represents your life from birth to death. On it will be recorded all the significant events of your life. My life-line is drawn below and although it is more complicated than most, it is basically similar to the life-line of most middle class women's.

Your life-line should start with your birth, continue on to the present and then project into the future for as long as you expect to live. You will see that my life-line goes to the year 100. This date is somewhat facetious, to be sure, but I do come from long lived stock. My grandmother lived to be 88 and two of her sisters lived to be 97 and 103 years old.

On my life-line I have listed marital history, child-bearing and child-rearing activities, education, paid work experience and personal interests. I have extended into the future those activities that I plan to be doing in my middle and old age.

## VIDAL S. CLAY LIFE-LINE

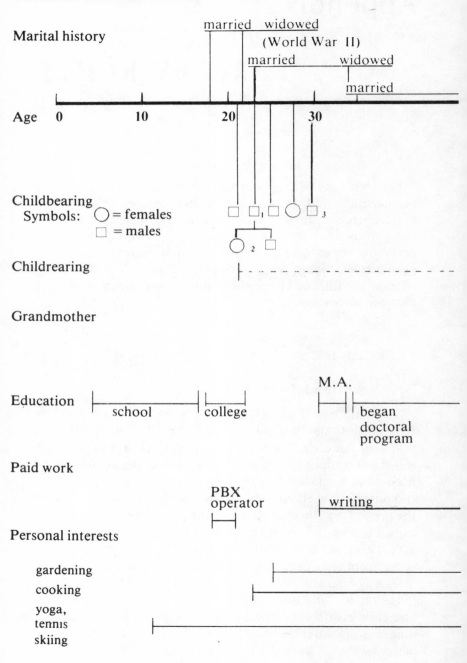

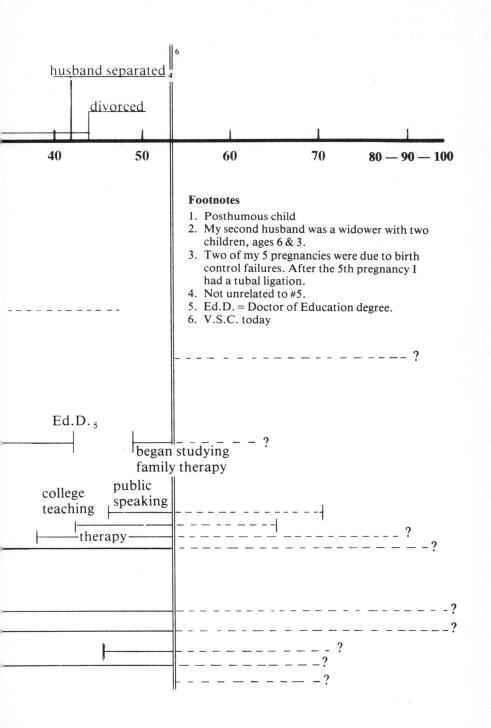

husband separated [4]

divorced

| 40 | 50 | 60 | 70 | 80 — 90 — 100 |

[6]

**Footnotes**
1. Posthumous child
2. My second husband was a widower with two children, ages 6 & 3.
3. Two of my 5 pregnancies were due to birth control failures. After the 5th pregnancy I had a tubal ligation.
4. Not unrelated to #5.
5. Ed.D. = Doctor of Education degree.
6. V.S.C. today

Ed.D. [5]

began studying family therapy

college teaching

public speaking

therapy

As you read my life-line you will see that I married early, at 19, and had five children in eight years. I was widowed twice, and each time I remarried a year later. I have been divorced. I reared a combined family of seven children, mine, his and ours, for nearly 30 years.

Educationally I completed my B.A. after I was married. I went back to college for my M.A. after the birth of my youngest child. I returned for my advanced degree, the Ed. D., or doctor of education, after I was widowed.

My paid work experienced includes a short stint as a PBX switchboard operator before the children were born. I didn't work for pay again for 20 years until I got my M.A. and began teaching on the college level part-time. I sold my first article to *Women's Day* after I went back to graduate school.

Tolday I am a woman on my own. My children have grown and left home. I have become a grandmother for the first time. I am again continuing my education in the field of family therapy. I expect to continue teaching until I have to retire, and then I will continue as a speaker, author and therapist as long as I am able. My father has set a strong example. At 81 years he still does research and publishes his work.

My personal interests include an interest in nature, gardening, cooking and athletics. These interests have changed over the years. I have always had a flower garden, but this spring I began an organic vegetable garden. In cooking, my interests now are in natural foods and eating less meat. I have always loved athletics and have played tennis and paddle tennis for years. Several years ago I took up Yoga. It seems to help the mind and body. Last winter I went to "ski-school" to learn to ski.

As you can see on my life-line, I anticipate continuing these interests, and no doubt I'll add some new ones in the years ahead.

Now draw your own life-line. Put on it all the events which have been significant in your life. It may help to think in terms of your education, paid work history, marriage, child-rearing, your personal interests and future plans.

Now study your own life-line. Can you see the years where you were busy with child-rearing? Can you see why you are not so busy now? How much longer will you be "mothering"?

How many years lie ahead of you? What are you going to do to occupy yourself fruitfully for this period of time? Will you be a full-time wife, mother, grandmother? You can expect to outlive your husband. What will you do after he dies?

Are you working for pay now? Do you plan to continue this work until you are 65? What will you do after that? If you are not working for pay now, do you want to work outside the home for pay or do you want to do volunteer work for causes which interest you? What skills and education do you have? Are your skills and education relevant today? Are they useful? Will you need more education and training before you develop a skill that you can sell in today's labor market? And in the future?

What interests do you have? Are they sufficient to make you feel good about your life in the years ahead? If they are not, can you use your interests to develop some paid work, a new career, or volunteer work for yourself? Will you be able to continue the interests you enjoy now into your old age? (We will look into your interests further in Exercise 3.) Study your life-line again. What are you going to do with the rest of your life so that it is satisfying and meaningful to you?

## EXERCISE 2

### Draw Your Personal Sociogram

In this exericse you will draw a diagram of your social world. You will draw what might be termed your social network, placing you in relation to the people you care about. These people can include, for instance, your mate, or partner if you have one, your children, their spouses and grandchildren if any. You may want to include your parents, your brothers and sisters, and their spouses, if you care for them. Consider your mate's family, good friends, people you work with etc.

Place yourself as a dot in the center of the page. Using the symbol of a circle for a female and a square for a male, then varying the size of the symbol according to your feelings for that person, place the people you care about on the page. For example, a favorite son would rate a large square and a sister-in-law you do not get along with, a small circle. Let the distance on the paper represent the distance these people are geographically from you. Thus a son at a University in England would be placed at the edge of the paper but his square would be large in size.

If you have a lot of people you care for in your life, it will help to keep them straight if you put their initials inside each symbol. You can put down as many or as few people as come to mind. You can list people who have died, if they are still very important to you. However, put an X through the circle or square to indicate that the person is dead. Here is an example of a sociogram. It is not mine, but that of a friend.

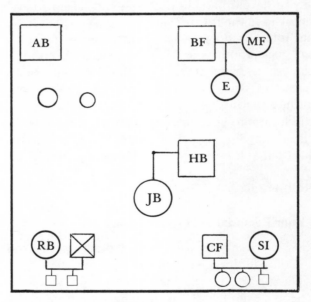

Make a diagram of your own sociogram.

When you have finished, study it. It is your life. What does it tell you? For instance, do you have a large social network? Or do you have just a few people who are important to you in your life? Are the people you care for close to you in terms of physical distance? For example, do they live nearby? Have your parents died and your children moved away?

Study your sociogram; think about it. What can you learn about your life? Can you realize anything new about yourself? Were you surprised by anything? Pleased, discouraged, disappointed? Is your life as it is now satisfactory or unsatisfactory in terms of having close interpersonal relationships? What changes can you make in your life so it will suit you better?

The first time I did this exercise, I suddenly realized why I had been feeling lonely and depressed. I was a woman alone and all my children had moved to far away places. Moreover none of my extended family, my parents, brothers or other relatives, lived nearby. I realized that I had few close women friends. I also realized that at this time in my life it was unlikely that I would make another committed relationship with a man. The odds are against it.

After pondering these insights I realized that nothing magical was going to happen to change the loneliness in my life. I understood that I would have to take charge of my life myself. I would have to create a new social network of good friends. I saw that is was up to me to make the effort to visit my children, realizing however that they are adults now and well-launched into their own lives.

## EXERCISE 3

### 20 Things I like To Do (Simon, Howe and Kirschenbaum, 1972)

Draw a line down the center of a page. Write the numbers from 1 to 20 down this line. Now, make a list of 20 things you like to do. You can stop at less than 20 or you can list more. It doesn't matter. They can be significant things in your life or small pleasures. Write them down as they come into your head. Order isn't important. If you get stuck, think of the seasons of the year.

1.

2.

2.

4.

5.

20.

When your list is complete, read it carefully and select the activity listed which you most enjoy. Put a 1 beside that activity. Choose number 2, 3, 4, and 5, recording the rating down the left hand side of the page.

Second, put a dollar sign ($) beside any activity which costs more than $5.00 each time you do them. You can vary the amount to suit yourself. What is important is that the amount of money spent is enough to force you to stop and consider whether or not you can afford to spend it.

Third. Place the letter A next to all activities you enjoy doing alone.

Fourth. Put the code N5 next to all those items you would *not* have listed 5 years ago.

Finally, put a star or asterisk beside each item that you will still be able to do and enjoy when you are 65 years old. Or older.

Now study your chart. What does it tell you? What can you learn from it? Ask yourself the following questions:

1. Which of the items listed do you like to do best? How often do you do your five favorite things? Do you do them regularly? Do you do some and not others, or do you do them rarely or not at all. Why? It is your life.

2. Study where you put your dollar signs. What can you learn about your need for money? Do you have caviar tastes? Can you only be happy with a cruise on the France or a box at the opera? Or can you enjoy things which cost very little money, or no money at all? Like taking a walk in the autumn leaves, for instance. Or watching a sunset. Most older women are poor. Will you have money in your older years? Will you need to develop activities which you can enjoy but which are inexpensive?

3. Check your A's. Are there things which you like to do alone? Many people confuse being alone with being lonely. There is a great difference between them. If you have a strong need to have people to do things with, it is something to consider for the future. Many older women are alone.

4. Where did you put your N5's? Have you learned to enjoy some new things in the past five years? A lot of people stop learning new activities when they are adults, but people can continue to learn all through their lives. A wise person has

said that each year you should add one new thing you like to do to your life. Certainly learning new things to do and enjoy is one of the excitements of living.

5. Look at your *'s. How many of the activities which you enjoy now will you be able to do when you are 65?

Study your list again. What can you learn about yourself?

Beyond these questions which I have posed, there are several more which you might ask yourself. Consider, Am I really getting what I want from my life? How will my life be in the future for me? What can I do *now* to make my life more enjoyable and fulfilling? What can I do now to make my life satisfactory for me in the future?

# BIBLIOGRAPHY

**A.** *Sources*

American Cancer Society, Inc. *Cancer Facts and Figures, 1975.* American Cancer Society, Inc., 219 East 42nd Street, New York, NY.

American Home Products Corporation. *Annual Report, 1973.* American Home Products Corporation, 685 Third Avenue, New York, NY 10017.

American Medical Association. *AMA Drug Evaluations.* Acton, MA: Publishing Science Group, Inc., 1973.

Angrist, Shirley S. and Almquist, Elizabeth. *Careers and Contingencies.* New York: Dunellen, 1975.

Barbach, Lonnie Garfield. *For Yourself: The Fulfillment of Female Sexuality.* Garden City, NY: Anchor Books, 1976.

Bart, Pauline. "Social Structure and Vocabularies of Disfort: What Happened to Female Hysteria?" *Journal of Health and Social Behavior.* September 1968.

Bockar, Joyce A., M.D. Personal communication. 1976 500 Newfield Avenue, Stamford, CT. 06905.

Boston Women's Health Book Collective. *Our Bodies, Ourselves* (2nd ed.). New York: Simon & Schuster, 1976.

Brody, Jane E. "Curb is Proposed on Vaginal Drug." *New York Times.* July 4, 1975a.

Brody, Jane E. "Experts Ask FDA Control on Estrogen." *New York Times.* December 21, 1975b.

Brody, Jane E. "Estrogen After Menopause No Bar to Cancer." *New York Times.* August 17, 1976.

Brown, Janet, et. al. *Two Births.* New York: The Bookworks/Random House, Inc. 1972.

Cerra, Frances. "FDA Chief Suspicious of Estrogens." *New York Times.* January 22, 1976.

Carson, Ruth. "Your Menopause." Public Affairs Pamphlet No. 447. New York Public Affairs Committee, 381 Park Ave. S., N.Y. 10016, 1970.

Chabon, Irwin, M.D. "The Menopause and Estrogen Therapy." *Journal of Reproductive Medicine.* Vol. 11, No. 6, December, 1973.

Cherry, Rona and Cherry, Lawrence. "Slowing the Clock of Age." *New York Times Magazine.* May 12, 1974.

Chittenden, George H. "The Privilege of Involvement." *Vassar Quarterly.* Spring 1975, Vol. LXXI, No. 3.

Clay, Vidal S. "Where are the Neighbors Bringing in Food?" *The Single Parent.* Vol. XVII, No. 6, July/August, 1974.

Clay, Vidal S. "Where are the Neighbors Bringing in Food?" *Pilgrimage Magazine.* Vol. XVII, No. 6, July/August, 197r.

Clevenger, Celia Faulkner. "Washington Opportunities for Women." *Vassar Quarterly.* Spring, 1975, Vol. LXXI, No. 3.

Connell, Elizabeth B., M.D., et. al. *Hormones, Sex and Happiness.* Chicago: Regnery, 1971.

Consumers Union. *The Pill.* Mount Vernon, NY: May, 1970. Pamphlet reprinted from *Consumers Report.*

Cook, Alice H. *The Working Mother: A Survey of Problems and Programs in Nine Countries.* Ithaca, NY: Cornell University, 1975.


Davidoff, Ida F. and Markewich, May E. "Post-parental Phase in the Life Cycle of Fifty College Educated Women." Unpublished Ed.D. dissertation, Teachers College, Columbia University, 1961.


Ehrenreich, Barbara and English, Dierdre. *Complaints and Disorders: The Sexual Politics of Sickness.* Glass Mt. Pamphlet No. 2, Old Westbury, NY: Feminist Press, 1973.


Gause, Ralph W., M.D. "Roundtable: Sexual Responsiveness in Women". *Medical Aspects of Human Sexuality.* January, 1970.

Goodman, Robin Reba. "Diethylstilestrol, Gynecology or Genocide?" *Herself: Women's News Journal.* April, 1974.

Gorney, Cynthia. "The Discarding of Mrs. Hill." *Ladies Home Journal.* February, 1976.

Gorney, Sondra and Cox, Clarie. *After 40: How Women Can Achieve Fulfillment.* New York: Dial Press, 1973.

Gornick, Vivian and Moran, Barbara K., eds. *Woman in Sexist Society.* New York: Basic Books, Inc., 1971.

Harrington, Stephanie. "Two Faces of the Same Eve: Ms. vs. Cosmo." *New York Times Magazine,* August 11, 1974.

Hartman, William E. and Fithian, Marilyn A. *Treatment of Sexual Dysfunction; A Bio-Psycho-Social Approach.* Long Beach, Calif: Center For Marital & Sexual Studies, 1972.

*Herself: Women's News Journal.* April, 1974.

Hirsch, Lollie. Personal communication, December 21, 1973. c/o New Moon Communications, luc. Box 3488, Ridgeway Station, Stamford, Conn. 06905.

Huber, Joan, ed. *Changing Women in a Changing Society.* Chicago: University of Chicago Press, 1973.

Hunt, Bernice and Hunt, Morton, *Prime Time.* New York: Stein & Day, 1975.

"In Menopause, Rely on Your Own Hormones". *Prevention Magazine.* March, 1970.

Irwin, T., *Better Health in Later Years.* Public Affairs Pamphlet no. 446. Public Affairs Committee, 381 Park Ave., S., NY 10016, 1970.

Johnson, Sheila K. Growing Old Alone Together:" *New York Times Magazine.* November 11, 1973.

Kaplan, Helen Singer, M.D. *The New Sex Therapy.* New York: Brunner/Mazel Publications, 1974.

Kaufman, Sherwin A., M.D. *The Ageless Woman: Menopause, Hormones and the Quest for Youth.* Englewood Cliffs, N.J.: Prentice-Hall, Inc., 1967, Popular Library.

Keller, Suzanne, "Ethics for the Future" *Princeton Alumni Weekly.* Vol. LXX, January 20, 1970.

Kelly, G. Lombard, M.D. "Look Better, Feel Better—Can Hormones Help?" *Vogue Magazine*. January, 1974.

Lang, Raven, et.al. *Birth Book*. Ben Lomond, Calif.: Genesis Press, 1972.

Lappé, Frances Moore. *Diet for a Small Planet*. New York: Ballantine Books, Inc., 1971.

Levine, Bernard B., M.D. "Estrogen and Uterine Cancer: Sale of Premarin Likely to be only Modestly Decreased." Research Report for Institutional Department of F. Eberstadt & Co., Inc. New York, NY.

Levy, John, M.D. and Munroe, Ruth. *The Happy Family*. New York: Alfred A. Knopf, 1966.

Lobsenz, Norman M. "Sex and the Senior Citizen." *New York Times Magazine*. January 20, 1974.

Machta, Phyllis and Jacobson, Michael. "Protein: The 'Buy' Word." *Nutrition Action,* Vol. 3, No. 1, January, 1976.

Margolius, Sidney K. *Health Foods, Facts and Fakes*. New York: Walker and Co., 1973.

Marmor, Judd, M.D. "Physiologic Factors and Emotional Disorders in Mature Women." From the Symposium on Physiologic Bases for Emotional Disorders in Women. The New York Academy of Medicine, Science and Medicine Publishing Co., Ayerst, 1973.

Mason, Karen Oppenheim, *Behavior Today*. June 30, 1975.

McCary, James Leslie. *Human Sexuality*. Princeton, NJ: Van Nostrand Co., Inc., 1976.

Mead, Margaret. *Behavior Today*. June 2, 1975.

Naismith, Grace. *Generation in the Middle*. A report by Blue Cross, Vol. XXIII, No. 1, Chicago, IL: Blue Cross Association, 1970.

Nemy, Enid. "Nutritional Problems of Women Discussed by Medical Experts:" *New York Times*. November 22, 1975.

Neugarten, Bernice L. "A New Look at Menopause: *The Female Experience*. Carol Travis, ed., Delmar, CA: CRM, Inc., 1973.

Oakley, Ann. *Woman's Work: The Housewife, Past and*

*Present*. New York: Pantheon Books, 1974a.

Oakley, Ann. *The Sociology of Housework*. New York: Pantheon Books, 1974b.

Ogle, Jane "Sex Begins At Forty." *Harper's Bazaar*. August, 1973.


Radicalesbians. *The Woman Identified Woman*. KNOW, Inc., P.O. Box 86031, Pittsburgh, PA 15221.

Ramey, Estelle. "She Is Woman." *New York Times,* September 24, 1973.

Raphael, Dana, ed. *Being Female: Reproduction, Power and Change*. Chicago, IL: Aldine Publishing Co., 1975.

Reed, Ann and Pfaltz, Marilyn. *Stop the World, We want to Get On*. New York: Charles Scribner & Sons, 1974.

Rodgers, Joann. "Rush to Surgery." *New York Times Magazine*. September 21, 1975.

Rorvik, David M. "You Can Stop Worrying About Menopause." *McCall's Magazine*. October, 1971.

Rose, Peter I., ed. *The Study of Society*. New York: Random House, 1973.

Rush, Florence. "Woman in the Middle." *Notes From The Third Year,* Old Chelsea Station, New York, NY, 1971.

Ryan, K.J. and Gibson, D.C. eds. *Menopause and Aging*. Summary Report and Selected Papers from a Research Conference, May 1971, Hot Springs, AK, DHEW Publication (N1H No. 73-319. Bethesda, MD: Public Health Service, 1973.


Schlenker, E.D., et al. "Nutrition of Older People." *American Journal of Clinical Nutrition,* 26, October, 1973.

Schutz, Dodi. "Have a Swinging Menopause." *Girl Talk,* March, 1971.

Seaman, Barbara. *Free and Female*. New York: Fawcett Crest Book, 1972.

Seaman, Barbara. "The New Pill Scare." *Ms. Magazine*. Vol. III, No. 12, June, 1975.

Seidenberg, Robert, M.D. "Drug Advertising and Perception of Mental Illness." *Mental Hygiene*. Vol. 55, No. l, January, 1971.

Shainess, Natalie. (Letter) *Drama Mailbag, New York Times*.

September 9, 1973.

Simon, Sidney B., Howe, Leland W., and Kirschenbaum, Howard. *Values Clarification: A Handbook of Practical Strategies for Teachers and Students.* New York: Hart Publishing Co., Inc., 1972.

Solomon, Joan. "Menopause: A Rite of Passage:" *Ms. Magazine,* December 1972.

Somers, Herman M. "Our Goal is Health, Not Medical Care." *University Magazine.* Summer 1975, No. 65.

Sommers, Tish and Guracar, Genny. *The Not-So-Helpless Female.* New York: David McKay Co., Inc. 1973.

Strom, Robert. "Education for a Leisure Society. *The Futurist,* April, 1975.

Syfers, Judy. "Why I Want A Wife." *Notes From The Third Year.* Old Chelsea Station, New York, 1971.

Travis, Carol, ed. *The Female Experience.* California: CRM, Inc., 1973.

Turnbull, Alexander C., M.D. "Estrogen Lactation Inhibition Linked to Thromboembolism." *Ob-Gyn News,* May 15, 1969.

Vanek, Joann. "Time Spent in Housework." *Scientific American.* November, 1974, Vol. 231, No. 5.

van Keep, Pieter A., M.D. "Aging and Oestrogens." *Medical Gynaecology, Andrology and Sociology.* Vol. 7, No. 3, 1973.

van Keep, Pieter A., M.D. and Freebody, Pamela, eds. *The Menstrual Cycle and Missing Menstruation.* International Health Foundation and the Transnational Family Research Institute, 1 Place due Port, 1204 Geneva, Switzerland. Report of Conference held November 11-12, 1972.

van Keep, Pieter A., M.D. and Kellerhals, J. "The Aging Woman." *Frontiers of Hormone Research.* Vol. 2, Basel, Switzerland: S. Karger AG, 1973.

Vizinczey, Stephen. *In Praise of Older Woman.* New York: Trident Press, 1966.

Weber, Melva. "Hormone Therapy." *Ladies Home Journal,* September, 1974.

Weiss, Kathleen. "Epidemiology of Vaginal Adenocarcinoma and Adenosis: Current Status." *JAMWA*. Vol. 30, No. 2, February, 1975.

Wilson, Robert A. *Feminine for Life*. New York: Wilson Research Foundation, Inc., 1964.

Women's Lobby Quarterly, Women's Lobby, Inc., 1345 G Street, S.E., Washington, D.C., October, 1975, Vol. 2, No. 1.

## B. Recommended Reading

### 1. Feminism

Ehrenreich, Barbara and English, Deirdre. *Complaints and Disorders: The Sexual Politics of Sickness*. Glass Mt. Pamphlet No. 2, Old Westbury, NY: Feminist Press, 1973.
Little about menopause here, but much is said about women and the medical establishment.

Gorney, Cynthia. "The Discarding of Mrs. Hill." *Ladies Home Journal,* February 1976.
How it is to be middle-aged and fall through the cracks of our social system.

Gornick, Vivian and Moran, Barbara K., eds. *Woman In Sexist Society*. New York: Basic Books, Inc., 1971.
Excellent collection of important articles on women.

Huber, Joan, ed. *Changing Women in a Changing Society*. Chicago: University of Chicago Press, 1973.
Excellent collection.

Rennie, Susan and Grimstad, Kirsten. *The New Woman's Survival Sourcebook*. New York: Alfred A. Knoph, 1975.
" . . . Goes far beyond cataloging the enterprises and services which have established the women's movement as an irreversible grass roots phenomenon. From politics to spirituality, esthetics to economics, sexuality to humor, the *Sourcebook* documents in essay and catalog form the *ideas* of feminism . . . " (from the Introduction)

Seaman, Barbara. *Free and Female*. New York: Fawcett
Crest Book, 1972.
Frankly feminist and a breath of fresh air.
Sommers, Tish and Guracar, Genny. *The Not-So-Helpless
Female*. New York: David McKay Co. Inc., 1973.
By the head of the NOW Task Force on Older Women.
A guide to social action.

## 2. Food and Nutrition

Benjamin, Alice and Corrigan, Harriet. *Cooking with Conscience*. CT. Vineyard Press, 1975.
52 simple, healthful, vegetarian meals based on protein
balance.
Goodwin, Mary T., and Pollen, Gerry. *Creative Food Experiences for Children*. Center for Science in the Public Interest, 1770 Church Street, Washington, D.C. 20036,
1974.
We can all learn from this book, and teach our children
good nutrition too.
Hewitt, Jean. *The New York Times Natural Foods Cook-
book*. New York: Avon Books, 1971.
Wonderful—Try it.
Jacobson, Michael. *Nutrition Scoreboard*. Center for Science
in the Public Interest, 1779 Church Street, Washington,
D.C. 20036, 1974.
Jacobson has developed his own rating system for the
nutritional value of food. Makes you think about what
you eat.
Lappe, Frances Moore. *Diet for a Small Planet*. New York:
Ballentine Books, 1971. Revised edition, 1975.
Margolius, Sidney. *Health Foods, Facts and Fakes*. New
York: Walker and Co., 1973.
A way to get the most out of the health food industry
and not get ripped off.
Shell, Adeline Garmer. *Supermarket Counter Power*. New
York: Warner Paperback Library, 1973.

## 3. Menopause

Cherry, Sheldon H., M.D. *The Menopause Myth*. New

York: Ballantine Books, 1976.

Hooray. A reasonable, responsible discussion of menopause by an M.D. who believes estrogens have been heavily overprescribed and should be used only for certain specific symptoms and only for a limited period of time.

Curtis, Lindsay R., M.D. *The Menopause.* Briston, TN.: Beecham-Massengil Pharmaceuticals, 1969.

Not recommended. This pamphlet and the one by Kelly are included here as typical of the materials made available to women in doctors' offices. This one is given free to doctors by the pharmaceutical company which makes an esterified estrogen tablet called Menest. This is written in a flip, cartoon-like way with educational chit-chat designed to educate women not to be afraid of menopause as drugs are now available. The pamphlet denigrates women. Some common symptoms of menopause are listed as "embarrassingly copious perspiration," also "senseless addle-headed anxiety."

Kaufman, Sherwin A., M.D. *The Ageless Woman: Menopause, Hormones, and the Quest for Youth.* Englewood Cliffs, NJ: Prentice-Hall, Inc., 1967.

An old classic. Does he have a new edition?

Kelly, G. Lombard M.D. *A Doctor Discusses Menopause.* Chicago: Budlong Press, 1959.

Not recommended. This antique is still being bought inexpensively by doctors and passed out to their female patients. The pamphlet has a fatherly tone to it. " . . . It will be comforting to have medical men in your life in whom you can place the utmost confidence." It recommends ERT under your physician's guidance. And, surprisingly, in a chapter, Perfecting Your Marriage, it recommends good sex.

*Menopause: The Experts Speak.* US Department of Health Education and Welfare, Public Health Service, National Institutes of Health. Publication No. (NIH) 75-756.

This little pamphlet is a simplified summary of the 1971 Conference on Menopause which was organized by the National Institute of Child Health and Human Development. The original report is cited frequently in the body of this book under the name of the editors, Ryan and Gibson, 1973.

Ryan, E.J. and Gibson, D.C., eds. *Menopause and Aging.* Summary Report and Selected Papers from a Research Conference, May 1971, Hot Springs, Arkansas. DHEW Publication (NIH) No. 73-319. Bethesda, MD. Public Health Service, 1973.

Heavy going for non-professionals. Out of print?

Solomon, Joan, "Menopause: A Rite of Passage" *Ms. Magazine.* December 1972.

Weideger, Paula. *Menstruation and Menopause, The Physiology, Psychology, the Myth and the Reality.* New York: Alfred A. Knopf. Inc., 1976.

Despite the title, this book is primarily about menstruation. It has interesting material in it about the physiology of the menstrual cycle, the sources of the menstrual taboo and the menstrual taboo in primitive and other cultures. As far as menopause is concerned, this book although published in 1976, is already out of date. It recommends ERT as "the primary cure for the menopausal syndrome." The only controversy about ERT that is mentioned is whether it should ever be discontinued. The recent studies linking ERT with cancer have not been included here. Otherwise, the information about menopause is good. Especially valuable is the linking up and tying together of the total female process: menarche, menstruation and menopause.

## 4. Middle Age

Hunt, Bernice and Hunt, Morton. *Prime Time.* New York: Stein and Day, 1975.

These authors view middle age through their own rose-colored spectacles. They speak of middle age as the prime of life and emphasize the real advantages that this time of life offers. I think they under-rate the problems that many middle-aged women face.

LeShan, Eda. *The Wonderful Crisis of Middle Life.* New York: David McKay Co., Inc., 1973.

Cheerful, optimistic. I couldn't get through it.

Sheehy, Gail. *Passages: Predictable Crisis of Adult Life.* New York: E.P. Dutton and Co., Inc., 1976.
A slick trip through the adult stages of life from age 20 to 50. It is written with a dash of psychology and enlivened with human interest case studies. Little is said about menopause though the male climacteric is discussed as a real change of life for men. What happens in the years after 50 is not considered in this book.

## 5. Physical Health

Boston Women's Health Book Collective. *Our Bodies, Ourselves.* New York: Simon and Schuster, (2nd edition) 1976.
In the first edition of this classic, the section on menopause was poor. This 1976 edition has been completely revised and expanded, and the section on menopause has been almost totally rewritten. It's a great improvement. The authors state clearly that ERT involves serious risks. The relationship between ERT and cancer of the endometrium is mentioned, perhaps as an afterthought as new studies on this relationship have only recently been published. Every woman should read this classic.

Haldy, Vera. *Being a Woman; a Guide to Your Body.* New York: Dell Purse Book, Dell Publishing Co., Inc., 1975.
Dell purse books can be bought very inexpensively at drugstores and supermarkets. They have a potential to reach a very large audience. It is pleasing to report that this small booklet is written from a feminist point of view. It stresses understanding your body and liking yourself. The back cover reads "For every women: your body is your home—this book shows how to feel comfortable in it."
Unfortunately the section on menopause is very out of date with recommendations for estrogen by injection which is described as being even better than the pills for menopause symptoms. Besides the sections on female physiology which are up to date, and good, there are sections on Eating Right To Feel Better, Good Health and How To Keep It.

Paulsen, Kathryn and Kuhn, Ryan A. *Woman's Almanac*. Philadelphia: Armitage Press, Inc./Information House Book, Inc., 1976.

The first 200 pages of this almanac are devoted to health, general, psychological and sexual. There is a lot of material here and most of it is excellent. The chapter on menopause is taken from the 1973 *Our Bodies, Ourselves*. Estrogen replacement therapy is recommended for severe symptoms but an editor has an added note about the new studies linking ERT and uterine cancer.

Rothman, Barbara Katz and Storch, Marcia L. *Woman's Body, Man's World: The Female Patient*. New York: Holt, Rinehart and Winston, Inc. (in press), 1976.

This book is still in press. Storch is a contributing editor on health to *The Woman's Almanac*. Rothman and Storch wrote "Update on Birth Control" in *Woman's Day*, June 1976, which was a balanced report. The new book should be good.

## 6. Managing Your Life:

*a. Jobs*

Abarbanl, Karin and Siegel, Connie. *A Woman's Work Book*. New York: Praeger Publishers, 1975.

The best book out on helping a woman to find a job. Good for middle-aged women.

Bolles, Richard N. *What Color Is Your Parachute?* Berkeley, CA: Ten Speed Press, 1974.

The best all around job-hunting book.

Irish, Richard K. *Go Hire Yourself an Employer*. New York: Doubleday/Anchor Books, 1972.

Also very good.

*b. Volunteer Work*

Loeser, Herta. *Women, Work and Volunteering*. Boston: Beacon Press, 1974.

A practical handbook by a feminist who recognizes that volunteer work has a valid place for women, and others today.

Somers, Tish and Guracar, Genny. *The Not-So-Helpless Female*. New York: David McKay Co., Inc. 1973.
Check Tish Somer's ideas about "valid volunteering."

*c. Survival*

Paulsen, Kathryn and Kuhn, Ryan A. *Woman's Almanac*. (See listing under Physical Health). This almanac is 12 handbooks in one. Besides discussions of health, it includes chapters on Education, Working, Business, Money, Legal advice, Politics, Handywoman, and Simple Pleasures. A fine collection. Expensive, but recommended.

Yates, Martha. *Coping: A Survival Manual for Women Alone*. Englewood Cliffs, NJ: Prentice-Hall, Inc. 1976.
This book is primarily a functional handbook for solving the important and practical problems connected with managing one's life as a woman alone. It includes chapters on managing money, finding and financing a place to live, coping with work, credit, your car, and repairs and maintenance of all kinds. A lot of information, much of it unfamiliar to most women but necessary to know, is presented in a clear manner. The chapters on coping with the emotional side of life as a single woman are less successful. Martha Yates is not a feminist. I found annoying the fact that in the chapter on coping with children, both girls and boys are called "he" throughout. Overall, this is the best book I've seen on dollars-and-cents, nuts-and-bolts management for a single woman.

# INDEX